D0086102

FREE Study Skills DVD Offer

Dear Customer,

Thank you for your purchase from Mometrix! We consider it an honor and privilege that you have purchased our product and want to ensure your satisfaction.

As a way of showing our appreciation and to help us better serve you, we have developed a Study Skills DVD that we would like to give you for <u>FREE</u>. **This DVD covers our "best practices" for studying for your exam, from using our study materials to preparing for the day of the test.**

All that we ask is that you email us your feedback that would describe your experience so far with our product. Good, bad or indifferent, we want to know what you think!

To get your **FREE Study Skills DVD**, email <u>freedvd@mometrix.com</u> with "FREE STUDY SKILLS DVD" in the subject line and the following information in the body of the email:

a. The name of the product you purchased.

b. Your product rating on a scale of 1-5, with 5 being the highest rating.

c. Your feedback. It can be long, short, or anything in-between, just your impressions and experience so far with our product. Good feedback might include how our study material met your needs and will highlight features of the product that you found helpful.

d. Your full name and shipping address where you would like us to send your free DVD.

If you have any questions or concerns, please don't hesitate to contact me directly.

Thanks again!

Sincerely,

Jay Willis
Vice President
<u>jay.willis@mometrix.com</u>
1-800-673-8175

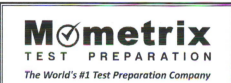

PMHN

Exam

SECRETS

Study Guide
Your Key to Exam Success

PMHN Test Review for the
Psychiatric and Mental Health Nurse Exam

Published by
Mometrix Test Preparation
PMHN Exam Secrets Test Prep Team

Written and edited by the PMHN Exam Secrets Test Prep Staff

Printed in the United States of America

This paper meets the requirements of ANSI/NISO Z39.48-1992 (Permanence of Paper).

Mometrix offers volume discount pricing to institutions. For more information or a price quote, please contact our sales department at sales@mometrix.com or 888-248-1219.

Mometrix Media LLC is not affiliated with or endorsed by any official testing organization. All organizational and test names are trademarks of their respective owners.

ISBN 13: 978-1-61072-573-6
ISBN 10: 1-61072-573-5

Dear Future Exam Success Story:

Congratulations on your purchase of our study guide. Our goal in writing our study guide was to cover the content on the test, as well as provide insight into typical test taking mistakes and how to overcome them.

Standardized tests are a key component of being successful, which only increases the importance of doing well in the high-pressure high-stakes environment of test day. How well you do on this test will have a significant impact on your future- and we have the research and practical advice to help you execute on test day.

The product you're reading now is designed to exploit weaknesses in the test itself, and help you avoid the most common errors test takers frequently make.

How to use this study guide

We don't want to waste your time. Our study guide is fast-paced and fluff-free. We suggest going through it a number of times, as repetition is an important part of learning new information and concepts.

First, read through the study guide completely to get a feel for the content and organization. Read the general success strategies first, and then proceed to the content sections. Each tip has been carefully selected for its effectiveness.

Second, read through the study guide again, and take notes in the margins and highlight those sections where you may have a particular weakness.

Finally, bring the manual with you on test day and study it before the exam begins.

Your success is our success

We would be delighted to hear about your success. Send us an email and tell us your story. Thanks for your business and we wish you continued success-

Sincerely,

Mometrix Test Preparation Team

Need more help? Check out our flashcards at: http://MometrixFlashcards.com/PMHN

TABLE OF CONTENTS

Top 20 Test Taking Tips

1. Carefully follow all the test registration procedures
2. Know the test directions, duration, topics, question types, how many questions
3. Setup a flexible study schedule at least 3-4 weeks before test day
4. Study during the time of day you are most alert, relaxed, and stress free
5. Maximize your learning style; visual learner use visual study aids, auditory learner use auditory study aids
6. Focus on your weakest knowledge base
7. Find a study partner to review with and help clarify questions
8. Practice, practice, practice
9. Get a good night's sleep; don't try to cram the night before the test
10. Eat a well balanced meal
11. Know the exact physical location of the testing site; drive the route to the site prior to test day
12. Bring a set of ear plugs; the testing center could be noisy
13. Wear comfortable, loose fitting, layered clothing to the testing center; prepare for it to be either cold or hot during the test
14. Bring at least 2 current forms of ID to the testing center
15. Arrive to the test early; be prepared to wait and be patient
16. Eliminate the obviously wrong answer choices, then guess the first remaining choice
17. Pace yourself; don't rush, but keep working and move on if you get stuck
18. Maintain a positive attitude even if the test is going poorly
19. Keep your first answer unless you are positive it is wrong
20. Check your work, don't make a careless mistake

Assessment

Subjective and objective information

There are two types of information that medical providers will receive from patients: subjective and objective. Information obtained through these means is what the health care provider will utilize in documentation. Subjective information includes what the patient tells you. This information is based on their description or opinion and is usually received verbally or through writing. Objective information is what the health care provider actually observes. This includes patient behaviors as well as any findings during physical assessment.

Interviewing the preschool child

In most cases, it is better to interview the parent and child separately. Children can usually give better information about what they are feeling, and parents give better information on their external behavior. When talking with young children, speak in simple terms and short sentences. Convey a neutral attitude. Most children between the ages of 1-4 understand more than they can communicate. Children may not be able to communicate absolute ideas. Assessing the child during play may give insight into real world experiences that the child cannot verbalize through questions alone. Play will often allow for evaluation of physical and cognitive development, adaptability, social and moral development, and coping abilities. It may give great insight into the child's perceptions of social relationships and family. Play may include drawing, dolls, puppets, dress up clothes, or use of modeling clay.

Patient history and data from multiple sources

During the admissions assessment, the nurse gathers information about the patient's history. The interview should occur in a space that allows for privacy, but it should not be isolated in case the patient becomes violent or threatening. Asking open-ended questions in a nonjudgmental manner (e.g., What problem brings you to the hospital?) is more effective than asking yes or no questions. Questions should focus on one problem or symptom at a time (e.g., Tell me about your sleeping habits.). Depending on the patient's condition, information may be obtained by:
- Directly interviewing the patient.
- Observing the patient's behavior and interactions with others.
- Reviewing previous hospitalization and discharge records.
- Interviewing family or caregivers ideally without the patient present so caregivers can speak freely. The nurse, however, must not violate the patient's right to privacy and should ask the patient's permission to speak with others.
- Interviewing police (if involved) and requesting a copy of police reports.
- Interviewing emergency medical technicians and reviewing their written reports.

Family assessment

When performing a family assessment, the health care provider will collect many different types of data relevant to the family's health and well being. They will evaluate the psychological and social functioning of the family and utilize this information to help identify nursing diagnoses. Information gathered may include the creation of a genogram, which is a graphical depiction of generations that identifies family members and their relationships. It includes their geographic relationship, age, date of death, and marriages. This picture should also include any known psychiatric disorders. By using the genogram, patterns can be identified. A family APGAR can also be used to help identify the family structure.

In-home medication list

When obtaining an in-home medication list, the first step is to ask if the patient has a list of medications or has brought current medications. If so, the nurse should review each medication, including the dose and frequency. If the medicine is available, the nurse should check the date on the medicine bottle as patients often keep medications for long periods of time and should assess the amount of remaining medication in relation to the dispensing date. If necessary, the nurse should ask the patient, family, or caregivers to provide information about medication, asking detailed questions about the drugs. Other questions can include the duration of treatment, reasons for taking the drugs, names of prescribing physicians, and the dispensing pharmacies. The nurse should specifically question any complementary treatments (e.g., vitamins, probiotics) and over-the-counter medications, asking about specific categories of drugs (e.g., pain medicines, antacids, laxatives, stool softeners, antihistamines) used both frequently and infrequently.

Normal cognitive development

Early childhood
Most pre-school aged children learn from what they see others do around them and thrive in environments full of stimuli. Whether a child is shy or outgoing, the sex of a child, and siblings and their ages are all factors that can affect language and cognitive development during this time. By age 2, most children begin to become aware that they are separate from others. They can speak simple 2-3 word phrases and are able to communicate simple needs. By age 3, speech becomes clearer and children can often form short phrases consisting of 3-5 words. They begin to engage in imaginary and social situation play. By their fourth birthday, the child usually has a vocabulary of approximately 1500 words and can easily form sentences using upwards of 6 words. Memory has increased and they can begin to recall stories or events.

School-aged child
School-aged children continue to have slow and steady cognitive growth. By age 8, most children have moved out of fantasy play and are more interested in real life scenarios. They have increased attention spans and enjoy working on tasks with friends or in groups. Following the rules and completion of these tasks becomes very important. They enjoy collecting things. They often make a best friend or establish a group of friends. They typically write clearly, however, they may reverse some letters. Their reading skills increase due to the fact that they can understand more complex stories. They are able to understand time in days and weeks. From age 9 on to adolescence, peer groups and social acceptance become increasingly important. They begin to understand and talk about the distant future. Day dreams or fantasizing are not uncommon. They have continued interest in reading and often enjoy fictional books.

Adolescent
As teens move through the adolescent years they begin to mature in their thought processes and develop a sense of identity. They begin to develop advanced reasoning and abstract thinking skills. Many adolescents have a greatly increased sense of self-consciousness. They often feel as if everyone is watching and judging them. A preoccupation with their appearance, behaviors, and feelings can develop. They begin to develop the ability to think about how they feel and how others

perceive them. Many teens develop a sense of immortality and participate in many high risk activities such as unsafe sex or reckless driving. They believe that nothing bad will happen to them. Confidentiality is also very important during this developmental stage, and they may be hesitant to share information.

Intellectual disability

Intellectual disability is usually diagnosed before adulthood. It is characterized by below average intelligence. These individuals are also unable to adapt to changing environments and need guidance in decision making. They may have self-care or communication deficits, and behaviors may range from shy and passive to hyperactive or aggressive. Those with associated physical characteristics or problems will often be diagnosed early. Diagnosis involves performance results from standardized tests along with behavior analysis. Intellectual disability can be classified from mild to profound. The following IQ scores determine classification: 55-69 – mild, 40-54 – moderate, 25-39 – severe, and <25 – profound. Safety is of utmost importance with these individuals. Depending upon the degree of intellectual disability, the ultimate goal for these individuals is achievement of some independent functioning within society. This can be achieved through caregiver support and education, along with promotion of coping skills and use of special academic programs targeted for people with intellectual disability.

Normal physical development

Preschool child
Children in early childhood range in age from 1-4 years. This age group makes great strides in their cognitive and physical development. By age 4 most children can run and kick a ball and get dressed and eat without assistance.   Normal healthy children in this age group develop mentally, physically, and emotionally at different rates. By age 2 most children can run, jump in place, and stand on their tip-toes. By age 3, the child has greatly improved fine motor skills and balance. They can perform tasks such as walk up steps, ride a tricycle, pick up small objects, and place shapes through appropriate holes. By the end of their fourth year, they can draw and cut simple shapes with scissors. By keeping regular checkup appointments with the pediatrician, many developmental delays can be identified in early childhood, and proper evaluation and treatment can be started.

School – aged child
School-aged children are considered to be between the ages of 5-11 years. By the age of 7, most children have continued slow steady development. Balance continues to improve. Most children of this age can balance on one foot, catch a ball, use simple tools, do some simple gymnastics, tie their shoes, and print words or short sentences. They start to lose their baby teeth and permanent teeth begin to appear. They may appear gawky due to long arms and/or legs. Older children from age 7 on to adolescence have greatly developed many of the fine motor and large muscle skills. Eyes reach maturity in both size and function, however, extended time viewing small print or screens can cause eye strain. School-aged children need approximately 10 hours of sleep per night.

Adolescent
Adolescence occurs between the ages of 11-20 years. Physical development occurs rapidly during the teen years and is commonly called puberty. It is during this time that secondary sex characteristics develop and the child becomes a mature adult able to reproduce. The physical changes that occur during this time include hormonal and brain development. In males the hormonally induced physical changes include development of facial, underarm, and pubic hair; changing of the voice; and penile development. In girls these changes include breast and genital

- 5 -

development, onset of menses, and increased growth of underarm and pubic hair. Both boys and girls experience rapid weight gain and increased production of oils and sweat gland activity leading to the development of acne. Brain development continues throughout the teen years. Neurons responsible for the maturation of emotions continue to develop. Many teens experience difficulties controlling their emotions or impulses, leading to bad judgment calls.

Adolescent developmental theories of Freud and Piaget

Developmental psychologists Sigmund Freud and Jean Piaget describe different theories on human development. Freud viewed development in biological stages of maturation. Adolescents experience the genital stage and experience a renewed awakening of sexual interest and exploration due to increased cognitive development. Their personality must adjust to cope with their new physical advancements. Piaget's theory has the adolescent entering into their fourth and final developmental stage – the formal operational stage. Once this stage is achieved, the adolescent will be capable of abstract thought processes and conceptual reasoning and be able to clearly discuss complex moral issues.

Age categories of the elderly

The elderly population can be divided into three groups. The age group ranging from 65-74 years are considered the young-old, from 75-84 are considered the middle-old, and 85 and older are considered old-old. There are many physical and psychological changes that occur as someone moves through these age groups. As this population increases in size, so does the number of those with mental illness. The mental health problems of this particular population are largely undertreated. Many rely on their primary health care provider to treat their mental health problems as well as their medical disease processes. Many of their medical diseases can lead to a loss of independence and feelings of helplessness, depression, and anxiety. Many leave lifelong jobs and lose friends.

Aging theories

The following are theories associated with aging:
- Biological programming theory: This theory describes aging as being pre-programmed and irreversible. The life of the cell is pre-determined by the DNA and is on course with its destiny.
- Cross-linkage theory: This theory describes the increasing rigidity that occurs during aging. Flexibility decreases due to increased collage bonds between many molecular structures within the body.
- Error theory: This theory describes aging in terms of malfunction and failures during protein synthesis that lead to errors within the cells. These mutated cells then multiply within the body.
- Free radical theory: Certain chemicals within the body, called free radicals, decrease the cells life span by damaging the membrane around the cell. These cells accumulate leading to an overall declining physical status.
- Gene theories: These theories describe the decline during aging as a result of the activation of destructive genes that damage DNA or the cells decline and they are no longer able to repair themselves. Some of these theories also consider the option that cells only divide a predetermined number of times.

- Immunological theory: This theory describes aging as a decline of the immune system. This decline can result in diminished ability to fight off disease or in turn become autoimmune in nature and reject its own cells.
- Stress adaptation theory: This theory discusses the physiological effects of stress on the body. Stress decreases internal balance and leads to a decreased capacity to fight off illness or disease.
- Wear and tear theory: This theory discusses the cumulative effects that normal every day insults have on the cell over time. The body is machine-like and the cells simply wear out from use over time.

Psychological theories

The following are psychological theories on aging:
- Erickson's stage of ego integrity: This is the 8th and final stage of development according to Erickson. He describes this stage as a time of life reflection. Completion of this task occurs when the individual feels a sense of fulfillment about their life tasks. The acceptance of this fulfillment will then resolve the battle between ego integrity and despair.
- Life review: This theory describes the process an individual undergoes when reviewing their life for purpose and meaning.
- Stability of personality: This theory proposes that an individual's personality remains consistent throughout life and that personality changes may be the result of physiological changes within the brain.

Sociocultural theories

The following are sociocultural theories of the aging population:
- Disengagement theory: This theory describes the withdrawal of the elderly person from engagement in society. This separation can be initiated by the person, society, or both and is considered the normal process.
- Activity theory: This theory describes the positive effects activity and involvement have for the aging population. The more involved and active they stay, the healthier both physically and mentally they will remain.
- Family theories: These theories place the family in the center of the aging population's well being. Their ability to move through the generational cycles within the family is reflected in both their emotional and physical health.
- Person-environment fit theory: This theory emphasizes the relationship between the aging population and how well they fit in their environment. As they move from young-old to old-old they may no longer feel safe or competent within their environment.

Changes with the elderly

Biological changes

As people move from the young-old to the old-old, many physical and biological changes occur throughout their bodies. Organs and tissues such as the kidneys, liver, heart, GI tract, and brain begin to decline, and some, such as the ovaries and uterus, fall into disuse and atrophy. Dysfunction of the kidneys and liver is of particular importance because these organs are responsible for drug metabolism. This population may also experience peripheral neuropathy, decreased reaction times, and decreased balance due to changes in the nervous system. There can also be a decline in the five senses. Changes in vision and hearing can affect performance on many of the assessment tools used to evaluate this population for mental health issues such as depression, delirium, dementia, or anxiety.

<u>Psychological changes</u>
Psychological changes can occur in cognition, learning capacity, and memory. These changes can lead to decreased continued development and can change relationships with family and friends. Many of the cognitive changes are brought about by a general atrophy in the brain. The aging process does not impair a person's state of consciousness, however, there can be a generalized decrease in concentration, attention span, and reaction times, leading to poor performance on many assessment tools. Learning may be diminished simply because the elderly person may lack motivation.
Memory loss does not go hand in hand with the aging process. Memory loss can occur for a variety of reasons such as disease processes, medications, substance abuse, or depression.

<u>Sociocultural changes</u>
The elderly may experience many social changes such as change in functional independence, employment, and social experiences with groups and friends. As the individual moves from young-old to old-old, many of the things they were able to do for themselves will diminish. This can range from fixing household problems to basic activities of daily living (ADLs) such as bathing and dressing. This population also enters retirement and daily life may become less organized and they may experience financial stress and anxiety. With retirement, this population may also have a reduction in healthcare benefits inhibiting them from seeking needed assistance. Debilitating medical conditions may also inhibit their social activities and they experience feelings of isolation.

Erickson's young and middle adult developmental theory

Erickson's young adult developmental theory encompasses ages 19 to 40 years. This stage describes the young adult as being confronted with their psychosocial development. They must learn intimacy and love or become isolated. Their ability to participate in a mutually satisfying personal relationship determines their successful completion of this task. The middle adult developmental theory encompasses ages 40 to 65 years. This stage describes the conflict between generativity and stagnation. It addresses the need of the individual to make things better for society's next generation. In other words, we are able to focus on the success of someone else. In this age group, this is commonly seen in parenting. If unable to move forward to caring for others, the individual will simply stagnate and be unable to move forward to the final stage of development in the life cycle.

Physical assessment

The physical assessment is a vital component in gaining a picture of the whole person. After a complete medical history has been obtained, a physical assessment should be performed. The person performing the exam should be aware of what is normal vs. abnormal. The information gathered during this assessment is objective. A complete physical assessment should progress systematically from head to toe and include all of the biologic systems such as neurological, cardiovascular, respiratory, GI, and motor movements. The patient's appearance, gait, muscle strength, coordination, eye movements and vision, hearing, and dentition, along with heart, lung, and bowel sounds should all be included. This information can be vital in helping to determine if any of the psychiatric problems may be biologically based, such as with some brain disorders.

A complete physical assessment involves the techniques of inspection, palpation, percussion, and auscultation. These techniques are usually performed in this order with inspection always occurring first. The exception occurs with evaluation of the abdomen, and then auscultation directly follows inspection. Touch, hearing, sight, and smell are senses that are all utilized while performing a physical assessment. Equipment such as a stethoscope, tuning fork, and additional lighting are all utilized with these techniques. It is also important to consider age and cultural influences upon the use of these assessment tools. Utmost respect should always be given to the patient.

Percussion

Percussion is utilized to elicit a sound by striking a body surface and is usually utilized to evaluate the chest and abdomen areas. The technique involves laying the hand palm side down upon the abdomen or chest and then firmly tapping the middle finger of the palm down hand with the middle finger of the other hand. The sound produced indicates the density of the underlying structure. The quality of this sound will indicate if the structure is solid in nature or if it is air or fluid filled. These sounds can range from tympanic, which usually indicates air filled, to dull, which indicates fluid filled or solid. Obesity can cause these sounds to be muffled and difficult to hear.

Inspection and palpation

Inspection involves what is directly observed during the assessment and is always performed first. It is an objective description of what is seen. It involves evaluation of colors, contours, and textures. It is often helpful to compare one side of the body to the other when evaluating normal vs. abnormal. Palpation involves using the hands to feel texture, temperature, consistency, pulsations, or movements. Deep palpation, which is performed after light palpation, involves the evaluation of structures below the surface for size, shape, or the presence of masses. Different parts of the hand are best for determining different sensations. The dorsal part of the hand is best for detecting temperature, and the lunar and fingertips are best for detecting sensations.

Auscultation

Auscultation is performed by listening to the sounds produced by the body and usually involves the use of a stethoscope. The cardiovascular, respiratory, and gastrointestinal systems are commonly evaluated by this method. The ability to distinguish different sounds will improve over time. The more assessments performed, the better the assessment skills become. Heart sounds can be difficult to differentiate. Normal sounds include S1 and S2 with abnormal sounds including gallops, murmurs, or rubs. Abnormal breath sounds can include rhonchi, wheezes, or crackles. Bowel sounds should be present in all four quadrants of the abdomen. Increased chest density or abdominal girth can cause sounds to be distant and difficult to hear.

Vital signs and lab values

Vital signs and lab values help determine a patient's baseline health status upon admission and then provide the ability to monitor these values throughout their stay or upon return visits. Vital signs include blood pressure, respirations, pulse, and temperature. Abnormal results can indicate the need for further medical evaluation and treatment. Common lab tests include CBC, BMP (chemistry), thyroid function studies, BUN, and creatinine to evaluate kidney function and liver function tests. Blood may also be drawn to evaluate HIV status or presence of hepatitis or syphilis. Drug levels and screenings may also be performed to evaluate current drug therapies or use of illegal substances.

> **Review Video:** Vital Signs
*Visit **mometrix.com/academy** and enter **Code: 330799***

Nutritional, appetite, and elimination screening

Nutritional and appetite screenings are valuable tools in determining if there has been any change in the patient's normal routine. Patients with depression may eat more or less than normal. With dementia, someone may forget to eat. Elimination patterns should be documented to determine a baseline of what is normal for the patient. Certain medications can cause a change in normal bowel or bladder habits. These changes can range from urinary urgency and diarrhea to hesitancy and constipation. Screening of these functions may also provide valuable insight into any eating disorders such as anorexia or bulimia.

Mental status examination

The mental status exam is a vital component of the assessment of the patient and is utilized by all members of the mental health care team. This exam determines what the patient is like at that moment. It should be documented so that later assessments can be compared to determine a change in patient status. The exam itself involves objective non-judgmental observations made by the staff member. It also includes what the patient communicates as well as their observed behaviors. Factors such as educational level and cultural beliefs can impact the results of this examination. The mini-mental state examination is a commonly used tool to assist in the documentation of the mental status examination.

MMSE

The mini-mental state exam (MMSE), also known as the Folstein test, is a commonly used assessment tool for evaluating cognition. It is typically used to evaluate for the presence and severity of dementia. The MMSE consists of a 30-point questionnaire that evaluates immediate and short-term memory recall, orientation, arithmetic, the ability to follow simple commands, language, and other functional abilities such as copying a drawing. In clinical settings, it is very useful to detect initial impairment or follow responses over the course of an illness and/or treatment. This tool establishes a score based on education level and age. This score can be placed on a scale to determine functionality of the individual. A total possible score of 30 can be achieved. A score of 24 or greater is considered a normal functioning level. The lower the score, the greater the degree of dementia or mental dysfunction. It is possible that simple physical limitations such as the inability to read or hear or decreased motor function may negatively affect the total score.

HAS or HAMA

The Hamilton Anxiety Scale (HAS or HAMA) is utilized to evaluate the anxiety related symptomatology that may present in adults as well as children. It provides an evaluation of overall anxiety and its degree of severity. This includes somatic anxiety (physical complaints) and psychic anxiety (mental agitation and distress). This scale consists of 14 items based on anxiety produced symptoms. Each item is ranked from 0 to 4 with zero having no symptoms present and 4 having severe symptoms present. This scale is frequently utilized in psychotropic drug evaluations. If performed before a particular medication has been started and then again at later visits, the HAS can be helpful in adjusting medication dosages based in part on the individual's score. It is often utilized as an outcome measure in clinical trials.

AIMS

The abnormal involuntary movement scale (AIMS) is an assessment tool that can be utilized to assess abnormal physical movements. These movements can often be the resulting side-effects of certain antipsychotic medications and can be associated with tardive dyskinesia or chronic akathisia. These motor abnormalities can also be associated with particular illnesses. Based on a five point scale, the movements of three specific physical areas are evaluated to determine a total score. These areas are the face and mouth, trunk area, and the extremities. AIMS has been established as a reliable assessment tool and also has a very simple design that provides a short assessment time. This allows it to be easily utilized in an inpatient or outpatient setting to provide an objective record of any abnormal physical movements that can change over the course of time.

Adult and pediatric pain scale

Because pain is very subjective by nature, the adult and pediatric pain scales are very useful ways to objectively measure how much pain an individual may be experiencing. This information can assist healthcare providers in monitoring their overall state of health. An accurate history is the first thing to obtain when you are evaluating pain. This history should include information such as age, surgical and medical history, medications, allergies, and baseline cognitive and functional status. There can often be multiple causes and locations of pain. Pain can be acute or chronic in nature. The adult pain scale asks the individual to place their pain level on a zero to ten scale, with zero being no pain and ten being the worst pain they have ever experienced. The pediatric pain scale is made up of pictured faces with expressions. There are six faces with the first face indicating a happy smiling expression and the sixth face showing a very sad frowning face indicative of a great deal of pain or discomfort.

BDI

The Beck Depression Inventory (BDI) is a widely utilized, self reported, multiple choice questionnaire consisting of 21 items, which measures the degree of depression. This tool is designed for use in adults between the ages of 17 to 80 years of age. It evaluates physical symptoms such as weight loss, loss of sleep, loss of interest in sex, and fatigue, along with attitudinal symptoms such as irritability, guilt, and hopelessness. The items rank in four possible answer choices based on an increasing severity of symptoms. The test is scored with the answers ranging in value from 0 to 3. The total score is utilized to determine the degree of depression. The usual ranges include: 0-9 no signs of depression, 10-18 mild depression, 19-29 moderate depression, and 30-63 severe depression.

Thought process descriptors

The following are definitions of thought process descriptors:
- Perseveration: involuntarily repeating a single idea, response, or activity. This can involve either speech or movement; however, it usually involves speech.
- Tangential: the topic logically changes to an entirely different topic; however, the person never returns to the original topic and does not answer the original question.
- Thought blocking: a sudden stop in the middle of a thought or sentence.
- Word salad: a string of words that have absolutely no relation.
- Circumstantial: speech that is unnecessarily and extremely detailed about a topic. The detailed information is usually relevant to the topic and the question is eventually answered.
- Flight of ideas: speech that rapidly and repeatedly changes or shifts from one fragmented idea or topic to another. These changes usually occur within one phrase or sentence.

- Loose associations: loss of the normal connected relationship of thoughts and ideas that makes speech and thought processes inexact, vague, and unfocused. Sudden shifts in topics or ideas occur without connection to each other.
- Neologisms: made up words that have no recognizable meaning. These can result from the blending of known words.

Thought processes

During an assessment the nurse should be alert for any alterations in the patient's thought processes. The patient can exhibit behaviors such as rapid movement between ideas, inability to speak directly or make a point, presence of disconnected ideas or topics, repetitive use of words or rhymes, or the use of made up words that have no meaning. The nurse should also evaluate the content of the words to help identify what the patient is trying to say. The patient may also fabricate stories or identify particular phobias, obsessions, compulsions, or suicidal or homicidal thoughts.

Risk assessment

Components
A risk assessment evaluates the patient condition and their particular situation for the presence of certain risk factors. These risks can be influenced by age, ethnicity, spiritual, or social beliefs. They can include risk for suicide, harming others, exacerbation of symptoms, development of new mental health issues, falls, seizures, allergic reactions, or elopement. This assessment should occur within the first hour of their arrival and then continue to be an ongoing process. The patient's specific risks should be prioritized and documented, and then nursing interventions should be put into place to protect this patient from these risks.

Evaluation for suicidal or homicidal thoughts
During a risk assessment two of the most important areas to evaluate are the patient's risk for self harm or harm to others. The staff member performing the assessment should very closely evaluate for any descriptions or thoughts the patient may have concerning these risks. Direct questioning on these subjects should be performed and documented. Close evaluation of any delusional thoughts the patient may be having should be carefully evaluated. Does the patient believe he or she is being instructed by others to perform either of these acts? Safety of the patient and others needs to be a top priority and carefully documented. If the patient indicates that they are having these thoughts or ideas, they must be placed in either suicidal or assault precautions with close monitoring per facility protocol.

A suicide risk assessment should be completed and documented upon admission, with each shift change, at discharge, or any time suicidal ideations are suggested by the patient. This risk assessment should evaluate some of the following criteria: would the patient sign a contract for safety, is there a suicide plan, how lethal is the plan, what is the elopement risk, how often are the suicidal thoughts, and have they attempted suicide before. Any associated symptoms of hopelessness, guilt, anger, helplessness, impulsive behaviors, nightmares, obsessions with death, or altered judgment should also be assessed and documented. The higher the score the higher the risk for suicide.

Fall risk
There are both physical and psychological deficits or abnormalities that can contribute to a patient's fall risk. Physical factors include weakness; lower extremity abnormalities that could

negatively affect gait or ability to bear weight; diarrhea or urinary urgency or frequency; or altered mental status due to medications, electrolyte imbalances, infection, or hypoxia. Psychological alterations that can increase the patient's fall risk can include dementia, delirium, other confusional states, paranoia, or suicidal ideations. Environmental factors can also increase risk for a fall. These factors may include lack of adequate lighting, lack of adequate foot wear, bed raised to a high position, unfamiliar environment, call bell not within easy reach, or use of restraints. All of these factors should be evaluated to provide the safest environment possible to prevent patient injury.

Background behavioral predictors of aggression and violence

During an assessment, the background history of a patient can reveal many different predictors of future maladaptive responses associated with aggression and violence. The history may reveal violent behaviors and rage responses, increasing irritability, or loss of control. Some examples of maladaptive background behaviors include cruelty to animals or children, setting fires or other destruction of property, drug or alcohol abuse, self directed violence such as cuts or burns on the arms, or juvenile delinquency. Many of these behaviors are evident during childhood.

Documentation of an occurrence report

Occurrence reports are utilized for facilities to track negative or averted negative events that occur within the facility. These reports are usually forwarded to the manager of the department who then forwards them on to risk management for review. They can be utilized to document occurrences such as patient injury due to a fall or any other cause; medication errors or averted errors; and inadvertent removal of IV's, feeding tubes, or other invasive patient lines by a staff member or the patient themselves. Any negative event or averted event should be documented on this form. Only the facts of what occurred are documented. No opinions or judgments about what the staff member thought might have happened are included. Any witness names, patient identification, and an exact explanation of what occurred are documented on this report.

Barriers to the patient assessment

Language or cultural barriers
Language or cultural barriers to performing the patient assessment should be evaluated by the staff member performing the assessment. If there is a language barrier, the staff member should be able to obtain an interpreter to assist with communication. Most facilities provide access to an interpreter at all times to facilitate patient-provider communication. The staff member should also be aware of any cultural beliefs or practices that may influence the assessment. The staff member should always strive to work within the cultural context of the patient. They should work to develop a sense of cultural awareness and knowledge. Each patient should be viewed as an individual with individual influences and beliefs and be treated with respect and consideration.

Physical and cognitive barriers
There may be certain physical or cognitive barriers to performing the patient assessment. An example of certain physical barriers could be if the patient has decreased hearing or speaking abilities or other diminished motor abilities. The patient may simply be unable physically to participate in certain portions of the examination. This information and an exact description of the patient's deficits should be documented in the record. Certain cognitive barriers may also be present. The patient may not be able to understand certain questions or be able to effectively communicate their answers.

Data collection on the prevalence of mental illness

The National Institute of Mental Health (NIMH) collects data on the prevalence of mental illness as well as treatment and costs. Most data are presented in graphs showing percentages while other data are presented as graphs showing rates per 100,000 population. Four primary categories of data include the following:

- Prevalence: Subcategories include serious mental health illness by demographics (e.g., age, sex, race), specific disorders, use of services and treatment, and specific populations (e.g., inmates).
- Disability: Subcategories include disability and years of life lost.
- Suicide: Subcategories include rates and causes of death.
- Cost: Subcategories include estimates, payers, receivers, trends, and comparisons (among the five most expensive medical conditions, which include heart conditions, cancer, trauma-related conditions, asthma, and mental disorders).

NIMH Collaborative Psychiatric Epidemiology Surveys combine the National Comorbidity Survey Replication, the National Survey of American Life, and the National Latino and Asian American Study to provide data regarding the distribution of mental illness and risk factors among various populations.

Resources for mental health professionals

The Substance Abuse and Mental Health Services Administration's (SAMHSA's) National Mental Health Information Center (NMHIC) provides a number of resources for mental health professionals. The NMHIC provides fact sheets and brochures, which can be ordered for distribution, on all aspects of mental illness. Training guides are also available free of charge. NMHIC also provides state resource guides for each state. Many fact sheets and reports are available for download directly from the website. SAMHSA conducts the National Survey on Drug Use and Health and provides data regarding the use of specific drugs, including prevalence, treatment, and emergency room admissions, with tables of detailed statistics provided by state. The Agency for Healthcare Research and Quality has been collecting data on health services used by Americans, including cost and payers. The Medical Expenditure Panel Survey has two major components:

- Household: This includes data on various health topics related to households, such as the use of medical care, payments, access, satisfaction, insurance, income, and employment.
- Insurance: This includes data from employers, regarding the types of insurance plans they offer.

Indicators of abuse

A great deal of information can be obtained through the nursing history. The nurse should always be aware of the presence of any indicators that may present a potential for or actual situation that involves abuse. Some examples of indicators concerning their primary complaint may include the following: vague description about the cause of the problem, inconsistencies between physical findings and explanations, minimizing injuries, long period of time passes between injury and treatment, and over-reactions or under-reactions of family members to injuries. Other important information may be revealed in the family genome, such as family history of violence, time spent in jail or prison, and family history of violent deaths or substance abuse. The patient's health history may include previous injuries, spontaneous abortions, or history of pervious inpatient psychiatric treatment or substance abuse.

During the nursing history the financial history, the patient's family values and their relationships with family members can also reveal actual or potential abuse indicators. The financial history may indicate that the patient has little or no money or they are not given access to money by a controlling family member. They may also be unemployed or utilized an elderly family member's income for their own personal expenses. Family values may indicate strong beliefs in physical punishment, dictatorship within the home, inability to allow different opinions within the home, or lack of trust for anyone outside the family. Relationships within the family may be dysfunctional and problems such as lack of affection between family members, co-dependency, frequent arguments, extramarital affairs, or extremely rigid beliefs about roles within the family may be present.

During the nursing history the sexual, social, and psychological history of the patient should be evaluated for any signs of actual or potential abuse. The sexual history may reveal problems such as previous sexual abuse, forced sexual acts, sexually transmitted diseases, sexual knowledge beyond normal age appropriate knowledge, or promiscuity. The social history may reveal unplanned pregnancies, social isolation as evidenced by lack of friends available to help the patient, unreasonable jealousy of significant other, verbal aggression, belief in physical punishment, or problems in school. During the psychological assessment the patient may express feelings of helplessness, being trapped, unable to describe their future, become tearful, perform self-mutilation, have low self-esteem, and have had previous suicide attempts.

During the physical assessment the nurse should always be aware of any indicators of abuse. These indicators may include increased anxiety about being examined or in the presence of the abuser; poor hygiene; looks to abuser to answer questions for them; flinching; over or underweight; presence of bruises, welts, scars or cigarette burns, bald patches on scalp for pulling out of hair, intercranial bleeding, subconjunctival hemorrhages, black eye, hearing loss from untreated infection or injury, poor dental hygiene, abdominal injuries, fractures, developmental delays, hyperactive reflexes, genital lacerations or ecchymosis; and presence of sexually transmitted diseases, rectal bruising, bleeding, edema, or poor sphincter tone.

Nursing observations

During the nursing assessment, observations made by the nurse can provide vital information about actual or potential abuse. General observations may include finding that the patient history is far different from what is objectively viewed by the nurse or that there is a lack of proper clothing or lack of physical care provided. The home environment may include lack of heat, water, or food. It may also reveal inappropriate sleeping arrangements or lack of an environmentally safe housing situation. Observations concerning family communications may reveal that the abuser answers all the questions for the whole family or that others look to the controlling member for approval or seem fearful of others. Family members may frequently argue, interrupt each other, or act out negative nonverbal behaviors while others are speaking. They may avoid talking about certain subjects that they feel are secretive.

Identifying and reporting neglect

Adults

Neglect of basic needs of adults is a common problem, especially among the elderly, adults with psychiatric or mental health problems, or those who live alone or with reluctant or incapable caregivers. In some cases, passive neglect may occur because an elderly or impaired spouse or partner is trying to take care of a patient and is unable to provide the care needed, but in other cases, active neglect reflects a lack of caring which may be considered negligence or abuse. Cases of neglect should be reported to the appropriate governmental agency, such as adult protective services. Indications of neglect include the following:

- Lack of assistive devices, such as a cane or walker, needed for mobility
- Misplaced or missing glasses or hearing aids
- Poor dental hygiene and dental care or missing dentures
- Patient left unattended for extended periods of time, sometimes confined to a bed or chair
- Patient left in soiled or urine- and feces-stained clothing
- Inadequate food, fluid, or nutrition, resulting in weight loss
- Inappropriate and unkempt clothing, such as no sweater or coat during the winter and dirty or torn clothing
- A dirty, messy environment

Children
While some children may not be physically or sexually abused, they may suffer from profound neglect or lack of supervision that places them at risk. Indicators include the following:

- Appearing dirty and unkempt, sometimes with infestations of lice, and wearing ill-fitting or torn clothes and shoes
- Being tired and sleepy during the daytime
- Having untended medical or dental problems, such as dental caries
- Missing appointments and not receiving proper immunizations
- Being underweight for stage of development

Neglect can be difficult to assess, especially if the nurse is serving a homeless or very poor population. Home visits may be needed to ascertain if adequate food, clothing, or supervision is being provided; this may be beyond the care provided by the nurse, so suspicions should be reported to appropriate authorities, such as child protective services, so that social workers can assess the home environment.

Diagnosis, Planning, and Outcomes Identification

Problem-based assessment and development of a problem list

Mental health patients often present with myriad health problems, so a problem-based assessment, focusing on finding a solution to particular problems can be effective. Problem-based assessment requires a thorough history, including questioning family members when appropriate, to develop a problem list. This approach does not preclude a complete examination, which might identify problems that the patient has neglected, but the focus remains on the problem list generated. The list should be prioritized to ensure that the most critical issues (e.g., suicidal ideation) are thoroughly assessed before less critical issues (e.g., occasional insomnia). Once a problem is identified, then differential diagnoses are determined. With some patients, there may be a combination of physical and psychosocial elements to a problem. For example, urinary problems may relate to depression, dehydration, lack of mobility, poor hygiene, medications, or disease. Appropriate diagnostic tests, further assessments, and interventions are completed as needed to diagnose and resolve problems.

Prioritizing nursing diagnoses and problems

Goals established for the patient
The plan of care is developed from information gained from the patient's interviews, history, physical examination, and medical records. Once a problem list is generated, the nurse must review and prioritize the list and establish goals for the patient, depending on the type of problem. Goals should be specifically related to the problem, measurable by some method, and attainable. Some problems (e.g., cardiac arrhythmias) can improve with treatment, so the goal is resolution of the problem: "Pulse rate should not exceed 90 beats per minute at rest." Other problems (e.g., chronic conditions) probably will not resolve, so the goal is preventing deterioration or further complications: "Patient should maintain current weight." Some problems (e.g., terminal cancer) cannot be resolved, and deterioration is inevitable; thus, the goal is palliation, ensuring the patient's comfort: "Patient should not experience breakthrough pain."

High, medium, and low and the ABCDE protocol
One method of prioritizing nursing diagnoses is to consider consequences (high, medium, low) if treatment is delayed:
- High (life-threatening): acute myocardial infarction and suicidal ideation
- Medium (delay may cause problems): malnutrition and manic episodes
- Low (treatment can be delayed safely): osteoarthritis and mild anxiety

Another method is the Advance Trauma Life Support (ATLS) ABCDE protocol, which is used to prioritize and assess in the event of trauma. The ATLS protocol steps include the following:
- Primary assessment of ABCs (i.e., airway, breathing, circulation)
- Resuscitation efforts to resuscitate and stabilize the patient
- Secondary review of the ABCs, adding DE, that is, disability and exposure/examination to provide additional information about the extent of injury
- Definitive treatment, such as surgery, as indicated

Maslow's Hierarchy of Needs

In many cases, prioritizing nursing diagnoses and problems can be accomplished by using Maslow's Hierarchy of Needs. Life-threatening needs and safety needs take precedence over others, regardless of the prioritization method used.

1	**Physiological** (basic needs to sustain life, such as oxygen, food, fluids, and sleep)	Risk for aspiration Deficient fluid volume Impaired spontaneous ventilation
2	**Safety and security** (physiological and psychological threats)	Verbal communication impaired Latex allergy response Death anxiety
3	**Love/belonging** (support, caring, and intimacy)	Risk for loneliness Anxiety Caregiver role strain
4	**Self-esteem** (sense of worth, respect, and independence)	Defensive coping Disturbed body image Post-traumatic response
5	**Self-actualization**	Health-seeking behaviors Spiritual distress

Absence without leave risk

All patients on admission to a mental health facility should be assessed for absence without leave (AWOL) risk, and those at risk should be monitored frequently, especially in facilities without good security. AWOL risk factors include the following:

- History of AWOL
- Elderly adult
- Suicidal ideation
- Substance abuse
- Inadequate family support
- Anger and hostility
- Fear or anxiety related to other patients

When a patient is believed to be AWOL, the first step is to notify security and to search the unit and facility thoroughly. Each facility must establish a protocol for notifications of AWOL. These may include physicians, nursing supervisors, family members, or police if the patient poses a risk to him- or herself or others or has been hospitalized by the court. Notifications may also include people who are at risk of injury because of threats the patient has made. Patients who have voluntarily committed themselves have a right to leave, but they should be followed at home to ensure their safety.

Learning disorders in children

Children with learning disorders often fall substantially behind their peers in regards to expected skill and academic achievement levels. These disorders are often classified into verbal and nonverbal groups that include reading, writing, and mathematics. Dyslexia, a reading disorder, is not defined by reduced intelligence. It has both genetic and environmental components and is a deficit involving the processing of the sounds involved in speech. Mathematic disorders appear to involve a dysfunction of the right-hemisphere of the brain. Medical conditions such as Turner's syndrome and seizure disorders can lead to right hemispheric dysfunction. Diagnosis of these disorders is often not made until the child reaches school and experiences a decreased performance. This group can often have low self-esteem and may need support to assist with these issues. Specialized educational training can improve functioning.

Autism in children

Autism is one of several different types of pervasive developmental disorders (PDDs). These children often do not achieve certain developmental milestones or these milestones are significantly delayed. These children are often isolated with an inability to socialize. Their communication abilities are often nonexistent. Autism is often characterized by repetitive behaviors such as echolalia, rocking, head banging, or extreme desire for rituals. An exact cause has not yet been identified, and medications have not been found to be an effective treatment. Early diagnosis and special education to help modify behaviors has shown some success. This is a chronic disease with disabilities ranging from mild to severe. There may or may not be associated intellectual disability. Many of these individuals require lifelong assistance and treatment.

> ➢ **Review Video:** Symptoms of Autism
> *Visit **mometrix.com/academy** and enter **Code: 507001***

ADHD

Attention-deficit hyperactivity disorder (ADHD) is commonly diagnosed in pre-school or school-aged children. It is more common in boys than girls. With this disorder the child has the consistent inability to pay attention, displays unruly conduct, and exhibits antisocial behaviors. It is characterized by hyperactivity, impulsiveness, and inattention. These behaviors may have been present since the child was very young, but since most children display some degree of these behaviors, ADHD may be delayed in its diagnosis. These behaviors may also persist through adolescence and may appear in some form into adulthood with less impulsivity as the child ages. Treatment for ADHD is long term and involves both the child and the family. Treatment should be comprehensive and include pharmacotherapy, psychotherapy, behavioral therapy, social skills training, or support services.

Diagnostic criteria
When evaluating a child for ADHD the first action should be to rule out any other causes of the behavior problems. The child should be examined for any possible medical problems such as seizure disorder, brain tumor, or infection. They should also be examined for learning disabilities, anxiety, depression, or significant life changes. Diagnostic criteria for ADHD are very specific. The child must exhibit at least 6 out of 10 symptoms of inattention and 6 out of 9 for hyper-activity. These symptoms must be persistent for at least six months and be inconsistent with their developmental level. Some symptoms must be present before the age of 7, and there should be evidence of social and/or academic impairment. Some associated symptoms may include low self-esteem, resentment towards others, decreased tolerance of frustration, and volatile temperament.

Communication disorders

Communication disorders impair a child's ability to communicate with others through speech or language development. These disabilities often go unnoticed and lead to delays in social and educational development. Examples of communication disorders may include stuttering, language delay, abnormal phonation, or mutism. Because their speech does not sound as expected, other children may tease the affected child leading to self-esteem problems and social isolation. These children should be encouraged to practice speaking for a period of time to aide in the improvement of sounds and comprehension. Mild communication disorders may not be diagnosed until adolescence. Specialized educational training and speech therapy may help improve symptoms.

Mood and mood disorders

The mood of a person is a long term emotional state that defines one's perceptions about the world and their place in it. It is an integral part of the personality. Variations in mood, such as sadness, anger, happiness, or anxiety, are a normal and expected part of life; however, these variations last a definitive period of time and do not affect normal life functioning. Mood disorders occur when these variations in mood cause distress and an inability to function normally. There are several terms that describe objective expressions of mood. These include blunted (reduced intensity of expression), flat (absent expression), inappropriate or labile (abruptly changing expressions), and restricted or constricted (minimally reduced in intensity of expression).

Adolescents

The most common mood disorders found in children and adolescents include major depressive disorder, bipolar I and/or II, dysthymic disorders, hypomanic episodes, and mood disorders related to substance use or medical illness. These disorders are more common in adolescents than in younger children. Mood disorders affect the child not only emotionally, but socially, and often lead to decreased performance in educational achievements. Manic episodes associated with bipolar disorders are often mistakenly diagnosed as ADHD. A thorough history, mental status exam, and assessment for self-harm should be performed. Support and education should include both the child and family.

Depressive disorders

There are several different types of depressive disorders. The first type of depressive disorder is major depressive disorder. This consists of one or more major depressive episodes. This type of depression is usually recurrent in nature with symptoms becoming progressively worse. The next type of depressive disorder is dysthmic disorder, which has milder more chronic symptoms than a major depressive episode. This is associated with depressed mood for the majority of days lasting at least two years with at least two of the following symptoms: lack of appetite or overeating, sleep disturbances or oversleeping, feeling fatigue, poor self-esteem, inability to concentrate or make decisions, and feelings of hopelessness. The final type of depressive disorder falls into the not otherwise specified (NOS) category and is a disorder with many depressive features; however, it does not meet the specific diagnostic criteria for a major depressive disorder.

Elderly

Many times the elderly population will not meet all the criteria or target symptoms for the diagnosis of depression. Many will only experience some of these symptoms and will often have associated physical illness or chronic disease processes. It is common for many of their symptoms to be somatic in nature. Treatment for this special population is very effective; however, it may take a longer period of time for the symptoms to improve. The risk for suicide is very high in this population. The highest risk groups include men and individuals over the age of 65. The highest risk group is actually those over the age of 85 years.

Children and adolescents

Children and adolescents experience many of the typical symptoms associated with depression. Children, however, usually will not experience psychosis. If this symptom does appear, they are usually not delusional. They are more likely to experience auditory hallucinations. Children are more likely to exhibit anxiety or somatic symptoms. They may be very fearful of separation from loved ones or complain of stomach or headache. Adolescents may appear more irritable and prone to conflict rather than experiencing feelings of sadness. Depression is more common in females than in males. Although the risk for suicide is high throughout the childhood and adolescent years, the highest risk is during the middle teenage years. Both children and adolescents of all ages should be closely monitored for any signs of this intention. Suicide is the third leading cause of death in teenagers.

Risk factors

There can be many different precipitating risk factors for the development of a depressive disorder. However, there are six particular risk factors that seem to occur more commonly than others. They include the following: a family history of depressive disorders, a previous episode of depression, a stressful life event, lack of a social support system, current substance abuse, and coexistence of a medical disease process. Major depressive disorders appear to have a strong genetic link for their development. The highest risk comes when a first degree relative, such as parent or sibling, has a history of major depression.

Major depressive disorder

Symptoms

There are several symptoms associated with major depressive disorder that contribute to the final diagnosis. These symptoms can include crying, irritability, anxiety, development of phobias, excessive worry, or panic attacks. These individuals can develop difficulties in maintaining personal relationships or experience sexual dysfunction. Many times marital and job problems will occur along with substance abuse. These individuals are at high risk for suicide and should be closely monitored for this potential. They may also experience physical pain and medical illness. Many times a major depressive episode can develop into chronic dysthymic disorder.

DSM-5 characteristics

The key DSM-5 characteristics for major depressive disorder include the following:
- The person has experienced a change in functioning from their previous state during a two week period of time. They are experiencing a depressed mood, extremely decreased interest in pleasure or normal activities, unintentional weight loss or gain with a change in appetite, insomnia or oversleeping, agitation or retardation of emotion and movement, fatigue, feelings of worthlessness or guilt, decreased ability to concentrate or make decisions, suicidal ideations or attempt without a specific plan, or frequent thoughts of death. At least one symptom is depressed mood or decrease in pleasurable activities.
- Significant impairment of normal social or occupational functioning.
- Symptoms are not explained by drug, alcohol, or medical disease process.
- Symptoms are not explained by another psychiatric diagnosis, such as schizoaffective disorder or bereavement.
- The person has never had a manic episode.

Adolescents

Depressive mood disorder is often characterized by a prolonged period of sadness accompanied by change in sleep habits, appetite, normal activities, socialization, and self-care patterns. Children are less likely to verbalize their feelings and often complain of more nonspecific somatic symptoms such as headaches or stomachaches. They may appear irritable, use alcohol or drugs, experience feelings of worthlessness or guilt, and may have suicidal ideations or thoughts of death. These symptoms must be present every day and last for 2 weeks or longer. Depression assessment tools and scales can also assist with diagnosis. A thorough assessment for self-harm is vitally important. Treatment goals include improving associated symptoms though support, education, pharmacotherapy, and/or psychotherapy.

Subgroups of major depressive disorder

Melancholic and atypical subgroups
The melancholic subgroup of major depressive disorder is more commonly seen in the elderly population and they can be misdiagnosed with dementia. They can experience symptoms such as the inability to experience joy or pleasure, exhibit an under-reactive mood, and can even move into a vegetative state. These patients must be treated with antidepressants. Electroconvulsive therapy is also a very effective treatment option with a very high success rate. The atypical subgroup of major depressive disorder is more common in the younger population and can be misdiagnosed with personality disorder. Symptoms can include overeating with weight gain, increased sleeping, overly sensitive to rejection, reactive mood, and experiencing a heavy sensation of the extremities. Treatment with SSRIs or MAOIs is preferred.

Psychosis
Patients who are placed into the psychotic subgroup of depressive disorder often experience the additional symptoms of hallucinations and delusions. They more commonly become bipolar and can be misdiagnosed as schizophrenic. They will usually have recurrent episodes that are often psychotic. Successful medication treatment options include the use of antidepressants along with an antipsychotic, such as haloperidol, risperidone, or olanzapine. Electroconvulsive therapy also provides a very effective treatment option for many of these patients.

SAD

Seasonal affective disorder (SAD) is when depression symptoms are often recurrent and seen during the winter and fall with resolution occurring in the spring and summer months. During the fall and winter the days become shorter and there is less sunlight. This pattern of depression symptoms is often associated with major depressive and bipolar disorders. Symptoms can include increased sleeping, increased appetite with carbohydrate binging, and associated weight gain. This disorder is thought to occur due to a change in the metabolism of melatonin. Light therapy is a treatment option and can provide some relief in mild to moderate SAD.

Postpartum depression

Postpartum mood disorders are divided further into three different classifications. They line on a continuum of symptoms from the least to the most severe. They include the blues, depression, and psychosis. Postpartum blues are short episodes that usually last less than 4 days. Symptoms include feeling emotionally labile and being tearful. These symptoms usually occur within 5 days of delivery. The patient should be reassured that this is a normal emotional response and will resolve over time. Postpartum depression usually occurs within 6 months of delivery; however, it can occur anytime between 2-12 months. Symptoms are similar to depression at other times during life and may require treatment. Postpartum psychosis is the most severe and can be further divided into depressed and manic categories. Symptoms will usually begin within the first month after delivery. Treatment is usually successful; however, many patients develop bipolar disorder.

Bipolar disorders

Bipolar disorders differ from depressive disorders due to the presence of manic or hypomanic episodes along with episodes of depression. There are three major subgroups of bipolar disorder. These divisions are bipolar I, II, and cyclothymic disorder. With bipolar I, there are episodes of major depression, mania or mixed episodes. With bipolar II, there are only periods of major depression and hypomania. A hypomanic episode is the same as a manic episode, except it lasts for at least four days instead of seven and does not lead to any social or occupational impairment. In cyclothymic disorder, there are episodes of hypomania and depression that have been present for at least 2 years; however, symptoms do not meet all of the diagnostic criteria for major depression.

Children and adolescents

In children with bipolar disorder, the hallmark symptom is intense rage. They experience this type of rage episode lasting for up to 2-3 hours. In younger children, many parents do not seek treatment for several years until the child becomes older and the behavior becomes more disruptive. For many younger children the first symptom exhibited is depression. Symptoms in children under the age of nine usually include labile emotions and irritability rather than more classic manic symptoms. However, as the child becomes older and enters adolescence, the symptoms become more classic-like and include abnormally elevated mood and delusions of grandeur.

Elderly

In the elderly population, bipolar disorder symptoms can often appear as a neurological or cognitive deficit, such as confusion. The onset of symptoms in this population is commonly associated with secondary mania and is due to medical problems, such as cardiovascular or respiratory disease processes. Secondary mania can also be caused by many of the medications used to treat chronic health problems. Late onset bipolar disorder is more commonly seen in women over the age of fifty or in men over the age of eighty. Successful treatment is difficult due to the presence of many chronic disease processes as possible causes.

Physical assessment

The assessment of a bipolar patient should always evaluate their current sleep patterns. This small piece of the puzzle can often give a good picture of the patient. The manic phase of bipolar disorder is often characterized by insomnia leading to emotional irritability and exhaustion, whereas the depression phase can lead to hypersomnia. Eating habits can also indicate a manic or depressive episode. Mania can often lead to decreased consumption of food and water resulting in malnutrition or dehydration. Body weight should be monitored. Any changes in sexual habits should also be assessed due to hypersexuality during mania.

Pharmacotherapy

During the acute phase, the main goal is elimination of symptoms and stabilization of mood. To achieve this, mood stabilizer may need to be used in polypharmacy therapy with antipsychotics or benzodiazepines if the patient is psychotic or experiencing agitation or insomnia. During the continuation phase, the main goal is to prevent relapse of the manic or depressive episode and to prevent the patient from swinging over to the opposite pole. This phase can last approximately 2 to 9 months and consists of close monitoring and continuation of the mood stabilizing medication.

During the maintenance phase, the outcome goal is to continue remission of the disorder and enhance quality of life. This phase may consist of life-long treatment with a mood stabilizer

Medication assessments

Medication treatment regimes for bipolar patients should be consistently evaluated. It is possible for the antidepressant medication used for the depressed episode to actually cause a manic episode. If this occurs the medication should be discontinued. Patient medication compliance is also very important. Many times the patients will feel as if they no longer need their medications and self discontinue leading to a manic or depressive episode. Patients should be well educated on interactions with other substances or alcohol and they may need to have regular drug testing to rule out substance abuse.

Possible nursing diagnoses

Nursing diagnoses for the bipolar patient can include both the physical and psychological aspect of their care. Possible diagnoses for the physical aspect of their nursing care can include: Disturbed Sleep Pattern, Sleep Deprivation, Imbalanced Nutrition, Fluid Volume Deficit, Hypothermia, or Noncompliance. Some possible diagnoses for the psychological aspect of their nursing care can include: Disturbed Sensory Perception, Disturbed Thought Process, Defensive Coping, Risk for Suicide, Risk for Violence, or Ineffective Individual Coping.

Mania

Mania is characterized by a distinctive period of psychophysiological activation. This includes a persistent abnormally elevated or irritable mood lasting for at least one week and is often a recurrent problem. Some of the associated behaviors can include euphoria, humorousness, inflated self-esteem, lack of shame, pressured speech, aggressiveness, excessive spending, hyperactivity, irresponsibility, sexual or social over activity, grandiose acts, or flight of ideas. This person can become dehydrated, malnourished, get very little sleep, or lose weight due to their state of hyperactivity. Many patients either feel happy and carefree or they may be irritable and argue easily with others. These patients have super inflated egos and lack of concern for others.

Assessment findings

Whenever a patient presents with mania, they should be assessed for any secondary medical disease process, such as endocrine or metabolic disorders including evaluation of thyroid function, neurological disorders, or presence of a tumor as a possible cause for the mania. Certain medications or substance abuse can also produce manic symptoms. Between the ages of 21-30 years is the most common time period for the first manic episode to occur. There could also be associated child abuse, spousal abuse, or other violent behaviors exhibited during a manic episode. These patients often have school related issues, occupational and marital failures, and exhibit anti-social behaviors. In patients who experience comorbidity, anxiety disorders such as panic disorder, social phobias and substance abuse are the most commonly occurring.

Stress and anxiety

Physiologic response

Sympathetic nervous system: The physical response to stress and anxiety occurs on a continuum from mild to severe. These responses are not controllable by the person experiencing these feelings and are mediated through the immune and autonomic nervous systems. The sympathetic nervous system turns on the physiologic response to stress and anxiety and readies the body to react. Under stress the hypothalamus acts to stimulate the pituitary gland to secrete a hormone that leads to increased cortisol levels. This increased production may lead to elevated availability of glucose for heightened cellular metabolism.

When the body feels increased stress and anxiety there is a release of epinephrine by the sympathetic nervous system. This affects the cardiovascular and respiratory systems by revving up their normal responses and readying the body to fly into action. In the cardiovascular system, the heart rate and blood pressure increase with associated feelings of palpitations. Blood is shunted away from non-vital organs, such as the stomach, intestines, and kidneys, resulting in decreased peristalsis and urine output. There is increased blood flow to necessary muscle groups to encourage a quick response time. Blood coagulation time increases. In the respiratory system, there is an increase in the rate of respirations and a decrease in the depth. Therefore, breathing becomes rapid and shallow and is associated with feelings of shortness of air.

The sympathetic nervous system usually leads to a decrease in blood flow in the gastrointestinal (GI) tract. This decreases appetite and movement of the intestinal tract. The neuromuscular system is charged up and ready to respond. Reflex time is increased and there can be some twitching or shaking of muscles. The need for sleep is greatly reduced, leading to periods of insomnia. The facial expression may be tense and the person may actually pace about. The skin may become flushed or itchy and there is an increase in sweat gland production.

During a sympathetic response to stress and anxiety there are not only physiologic responses, there are also associated behavioral and cognitive responses. The person may appear anxious. They may have uncontrolled muscle movements, restlessness, fast speech, avoidance, or startle easily. These reactions can lead to ineffective interpersonal communication or social withdrawal. Cognitive functioning can also be affected by stress and anxiety. The person might appear distracted or unable to concentrate, forgetful, confused, or make errors in judgment not normally seen. They may also experience flashbacks or have frightening hallucinations.

Parasympathetic nervous system: In most individuals the sympathetic nervous system takes over during a stress or anxiety response initiating the fight or flight response. However, in some individuals, the parasympathetic nervous system can dominate during this time. The associated symptoms often have the opposite effect of what is seen when the sympathetic nervous system is in control. Cardiovascular responses can include decreased blood pressure and heart rate, feelings of faintness or actual fainting. There can also be an increased need to urinate along with feelings of abdominal pain, nausea, and diarrhea.

Generalized anxiety disorder

Generalized anxiety disorder can be very insidious and occurs when an individual consistently experiences excessive anxiety and worry. This anxiety and worry will be present almost every day and lasts for a period of at least six months. The worry and anxiety will be uncontrollable, intrusive, and not related to any medical disease process. It will pertain to real-life events, situations, or circumstances and may occur along with mild depression symptoms. The individual will also experience 3 or more of the following symptoms: fatigue, inability to concentrate, irritability, insomnia, restlessness, loosing thought processes or going blank, and muscle tension. The continued anxiety and worry will eventually affect daily functioning and cause social and occupational disturbances.

<u>Comorbidities</u>

Individuals with generalized anxiety disorder (GAD) will often have other mental health disorders. When a person has more than one psychological disorder occurring at the same time, these disorders are considered to be comorbid. Most patients suffering from GAD will have at least one more psychiatric diagnosis. The most common comorbid disorders can include major depressive disorder, social or specific phobias, panic disorder, and dysthymic disorder. It is also common for these individuals to have substance abuse problems, and they may look to alcohol or barbiturates to help control their symptoms of anxiety.

Anxiety

Anxiety is a human emotion and experience that everyone has at some point during their life. Feelings of uncertainty, helplessness, isolation, alienation, and insecurity can all be experienced during an anxiety response. Many times anxiety occurs without a specific known object or source. It can occur because of the unknown. Anxiety occurs throughout the life cycle and therefore anxiety disorders can affect people of all ages. Populations that are most commonly affected include women, smokers, people under the age of 45, individuals that are separated or divorced, victims of abuse, and people in the lower socioeconomic groups. An individual can have one single anxiety disorder, experience more than one anxiety disorder, or have other mental health disorders all occurring at the same time.

Physical symptoms

Anxiety produces a very physical response and affects the largest body systems, such as cardiovascular, respiratory, GI, neuromuscular, urinary tract, and skin. Symptoms vary and can increase upon a continuum depending upon the level of anxiety the person is experiencing. Cardiovascular symptoms can include palpitation, tachycardia, hypertension, feeling faint or actually fainting, hypotension, or bradycardia. Respiratory symptoms can include tachypnea, shortness of breath, chest pressure, shallow respirations, or choking sensation. GI symptoms can include revulsion toward food, nausea, diarrhea, and abdominal pain or discomfort. Even though anxiety occurs psychologically, it can produce extreme physical responses from the neuromuscular, urinary tract, and skin. These symptoms can range from mild to severe depending upon the degree of anxiety the person is experiencing. Neuromuscular symptoms can include hyperreflexia, being easily startled, eyelid twitching, inability to sleep, shaking, fidgeting, pacing, wobbly legs, or clumsy movements. Urinary tract symptoms can include increased frequency and sensation of need to urinate. Skin symptoms can include flushed face, sweaty palms, itching, sensations of being hot and/or cold, pale facial coloring, or diaphoresis.

Levels

There are four main levels of anxiety that were named by Peplau. They are as follows:

- Mild anxiety - This is associated with normal tensions of everyday life. It can increase awareness and motivate learning and creativity.
- Moderate anxiety – This occurs when the individual narrows their field of perception and focuses on the immediate problem. This level decreases the perceptual field; however, the person can tend to other tasks if directed.
- Severe anxiety – This leads to a markedly reduced field of perception and the person focuses only on the details of the problem. All energy is directed at relieving the anxiety and the person can only perform other tasks under significant persuasion.
- Panic – This is the most extreme level of anxiety and associated with feelings of dread and terror. The individual is unable to perform any other tasks no matter how strongly they are persuaded to do so. This level can be life threatening with complete disorganization of thought occurring.

<u>Behavioral and affective responses</u>
Behavioral and affective symptoms along with a multitude of physical symptoms are observable in the anxious patient. The effects of these responses can affect the person experiencing the anxiety along with their relationships with others. Some behavioral responses can include restlessness and physical tension, hypervigilance, rapid speech, social or relationship withdrawal, decreased coordination, avoidance, or flight. Affective responses are the patient's emotional reactions and can be described subjectively by the individual. Patients may describe symptoms such as edginess, impatience, tension, nervousness, fear, frustration, jitteriness, or helplessness.

<u>Cognitive responses</u>
Anxiety not only produces physical and emotional symptoms, but it can also greatly affect the individual's intellectual abilities. Cognitive responses to anxiety occur in three main categories. These include sensory-perceptual, thought difficulties, and conceptualization. Responses that affect the patient's sensory-perceptual fields can include feeling that their mind is unclear or clouded, objects seem indistinct, surreal environment, increased self-consciousness, or hypervigilance. Thinking difficulties can include inability to remember important information, confusion, inability to focus thoughts or attention, easily distracted, blocking thoughts, difficulty with reasoning, tunnel vision, or loss of objectivity. Conceptual difficulties can include the fear of loss of control, inability to cope, potential physical injury, developing a mental disorder, or receiving a negative evaluation. The patient may have cognitive distortion, protruding scary visual images, or uncontrollable repetition of fearful thoughts.

Specific and social phobias

Anxiety disorders also include specific and social phobias. Specific phobias involve unreasonable fears of a specific object or situation. Some examples of these phobias include the fear of flying, heights, enclosed spaced, or spiders. When the individual is placed in the feared situation, there is a marked anxiety reaction. Social phobias involve an irrational fear of social interactions with strangers. This could also include a fear of having to speak or perform in front of others. They fear that they will be humiliated or greatly criticized by others. In both specific and social phobias, the person often is aware that their fear is unreasonable; however, they cannot control their anxiety level. Behaviors are often modified to prevent exposure to the feared situation.

Panic disorder

A panic disorder is a chronically occurring mental health condition. It will have periods of exacerbations, such as a panic attacks, and periods of calm and remission. After a panic attack, the person will experience fear about having another panic attack lasting for at least one month. It can occur with or without agoraphobia. Panic disorders can also lead to the development of other phobias, such as social phobias, or target specific phobias. The hallmark symptom of panic disorder is recurrent panic attacks with behavioral changes occurring due to these attacks.

Panic disorder with agoraphobia

Panic disorder with agoraphobia meets all the criteria for any panic disorder; however, the patient also experiences fear and anxiety about being in a location or situation in which escape would be difficult or help would not be readily available during a panic attack. Examples of these situations can include going outside the house, being in a crowded room, riding in a transportation vehicle, or crossing a bridge. The person would avoid these types of situations if at all possible. If they have no choice but to be in this situation, they would endure great stress and usually require the presence of a support person.

OCD

Anxiety disorders also include the diagnosis of obsessive-compulsive disorder (OCD). OCD involves either obsessions or compulsions that are persistent impulses or thoughts that are uncontrollable by the person. These thoughts lead to an abnormally elevated anxiety response. Some examples of obsessions can include fear of dirt, germs, robbery, contracting a medical disease, unintentional discarding of important information, having images of a sexual nature, or things not being symmetrical or completed. Compulsions are when the individual is driven to perform certain repetitive behaviors in ritualistic order with the outcome being resolution of the anxiety caused by the obsession. Some examples of compulsive repetitive behaviors can include hand washing, checking locks, counting objects found routinely within their normal day, hoarding, ordering or arranging items, or saying words silently.

Comorbidities
When an individual has two or more disorders occurring at the same time, these disorders are considered to share comorbidity. Obsessive-compulsive disorder (OCD) is often found sharing comorbidity with other psychological disorders. Many times individuals with OCD also have Tourette's syndrome, depression, panic attacks, mood disorders, social and specific phobias, eating disorders, or personality disorders. It has been found that Tourette's syndrome and OCD actually cause similar brain dysfunctions. Depression is commonly seen in patients suffering from OCD due to the isolating effects it can have upon their lifestyle. It is also common for these individuals to have substance abuse problems due to the fact that they are trying to self medicate to solve their struggles with OCD.

Acute stress disorder

Acute stress disorder also falls under the umbrella of anxiety disorders and shares some similar defining characteristics to post traumatic stress disorder. Both occur when an individual has been exposed to a traumatic even that was witnessed, experienced, or simply confronted with a potential life threatening event that could have affected the person themselves or others around them. During this event the person experienced extreme fear, helplessness, or horror. In acute stress disorder, the response post-event differs from post traumatic stress syndrome. After the event, the person will experience at least three of the following symptoms: disassociation, reduced awareness of surroundings, dissociation amnesia, derealization, or depersonalization. These individuals will have experienced unwanted recall or flashbacks of the event and will experience social and occupational dysfunction as a result of avoidance behaviors. The symptoms last 2 days to 4 weeks and occur within one month of the event.

Post traumatic stress disorder

An individual who suffers from post traumatic stress disorder has been exposed to a traumatic event. This event could have been witnessed, experienced, or they could have simply been confronted with a potential traumatic event that could have caused death or severe injury to themselves or others around them. During the exposure to this event, the person would have experienced extreme fear, helplessness, or horror. They often re-experience the event through nightmares or unwanted intrusive memories. They often experience unexpected and unwanted severe psychological reactions when a situation or cue triggers a memory or they are placed in a situation similar to the traumatic event. The person will modify all behaviors to avoid any situations where an unwanted anxiety response could occur. They often develop a generalized numbed response to many situations. If symptoms persist longer than 3 months, then the person is considered to have chronic post traumatic stress disorder.

Personality disorder

A personality disorder is a fixed and enduring set pattern or traits of behavior that deviates from expected behaviors within a culture. This disorder inhibits the individual's ability to have meaningful interpersonal relationships, be fulfilled, or enjoy life. Onset usually occurs during adolescence or early adulthood. A personality disorder is an attitude directed toward the whole world including ones own self. This attitude is expressed through thoughts, feelings, and behaviors. Many times the behaviors will become less extreme as the person gets older.

DSM-5 classification groupings
The DSM-5 has grouped personality disorders into three main classifications. These are clusters A, B, and C. Cluster A includes disorders that characterize odd or eccentric behaviors and have a tendency for social and/or emotional withdrawal. Cluster B includes disorders that are erratic, highly emotional, dramatic, and impulsive in nature. Cluster C includes disorders that produce predominantly fearful or anxious symptoms.

Cluster A: The classification of Cluster A for personality disorders includes the diagnoses of the following types of personalities: paranoid, schizoid, and schizotypal. The paranoid individual is very distrustful and suspicious of others. They believe that other people are up to no good, are keeping secrets, and may intend to harm them. There is usually no basis or evidence to support this belief. The schizoid individual exhibits a consistent social detachment. Many of their behaviors indicate a restricted emotional response and can include appearing cold and indifferent, having no desire for close personal relationships, having no desire for intimacy, choosing solidarity over socializing, and usually having no close friends or relatives. The schizotypal individual may exhibit odd eccentric behaviors or express magical beliefs. They usually have no close friends or relatives and are socially isolated, believing that they are not accepted by others. They may have paranoid ideations and experience discomfort or acute anxiety when in social situations.

Cluster B: The classification of Cluster B for personality disorders includes the diagnoses of antisocial, borderline, histrionic, and narcissistic personality types. The antisocial individual exhibits a blatant disregard for other people. They frequently lie, manipulate, exploit, and commit illegal acts. The borderline individual has a markedly unstable self-image. They are very impulsive, self-destructive, have unstable and intense interpersonal relationships, mood instability, inappropriate and intense anger, and may have recurrent suicidal or self-mutilating behaviors. The histrionic individual is extremely emotional and desires to be the center of attention. They often perform attention seeking behaviors and have frequent intense short-lived relationships. The narcissistic individual has a great sense of self-importance and is often arrogant. They lack empathy for others and can be exploitative and manipulative.

Cluster C: The classification of Cluster C for personality disorders includes the diagnoses of avoidant, dependent, and obsessive-compulsive personality types. The avoidant individual does not participate in social or occupational situations that require much interaction with other people. They are very sensitive to negative criticism or rejection and feel as though they are inadequate. The dependent individual has very low self-esteem and will be submissive and dependent in behaviors and relationships. They do not like to be alone and they will seek out a new relationship as soon as one ends. The obsessive-compulsive individual will have an extreme preoccupation with minute details, perfectionism, and control. They will often exhibit cold, unfeeling, and superior attitudes towards others.

Anorexia nervosa

Anorexia nervosa is an illness that is associated with an eating disorder. It is most commonly seen in females and onset usually occurs between 13 and 20 years of age; however, it can occur in any age group. The symptoms can be very insidious and years can go by before the individual receives any treatment. The patient will refuse to maintain an adequate body weight due to a distorted body image or fear of becoming fat. This illness is usually chronic and requires a lifetime of monitoring. Many times even though the individual will maintain a normal body weight, they will still be preoccupied with food and may develop subsequent eating disorders such as bulimia nervosa or continue to have other psychiatric disorders and symptoms.

Physical findings
Many of the characteristic physical findings associated with anorexia nervosa are a result of malnutrition and starvation. This disease affects all of the major body systems, such as cardiovascular, GI, musculoskeletal, skin, reproductive, and metabolic. Symptoms can include fatigue or excessive energy, constipation or diarrhea, abdominal pain due to bloating, sensitivity to cold temperatures, emaciated appearance, hypotension, low body temperature, osteoporosis, dry skin, brittle nails, hair loss, amenorrhea or irregular menstrual cycles, bradycardia or other life threatening cardiac arrhythmias, seizures, edema of hands or feet, hypertrophy of salivary glands, dental enamel erosion, and scars on dorsum of hand from the teeth due to induced vomiting.

Diagnostic criteria
The diagnostic characteristics for anorexia nervosa include the following:
- Refusal to maintain a minimal normal body weight.
- Extreme fear of becoming fat.
- Disturbed perception of body weight or shape.
- Denial of low body weight and high priority placed on weight or body shape in regards to self-evaluation.
- Amenorrhea for at least 3 consecutive menstrual cycles.
- Restrictive type does not involve in binge or purge behaviors.
- Binge eating and purging type regularly involved in binge or purge behaviors.

Laboratory findings
Many of the abnormal lab findings are associated with the malnutrition and starvation that occurs with anorexia nervosa. Some of the common lab findings can include mild anemia; leucopenia; elevated BUN from dehydration; high cholesterol; hypoglycemia; elevated liver function studies; thrombocytopenia; electrolyte imbalances, particularly hypokalemia (low potassium); metabolic alkalosis or acidosis; hypothyroidism; or decreased estrogen, LH, and FSH hormone levels. In the more severe cases the patient can develop metabolic encephalopathy or increased ventricular/brain ratio resulting due to the complications of starvation. This disease can result in death.

Psychological symptoms
Patients with anorexia nervosa exhibit many mental health symptoms. They commonly have comorbidity with depression and dysthymia. They may be irritable, have sleep disturbances, a lack

of interest in sex, and withdrawal from social interactions. They will be obsessed with the thought of food and may also have other obsessive-compulsive tendencies that may or may not involve food. They are very self conscious about eating in public, seek to have total control over their environment, and commonly have panic attacks or other phobias. They often have very rigid views and opinions, are perfectionists, may not express their emotions, and can be at high risk for suicide.

Nursing interventions
Patients that are hospitalized for anorexia nervosa are usually severely malnourished and require monitoring of their food consumption and activities. Their lives often depend upon their bodies receiving nutrition and hydration. These patients should participate in psychotherapy and be allowed to verbalize their feelings and anxieties about food consumption and weight gain. Intake of meals and snacks should be documented. Food substitutions should not be allowed and caffeinated drinks limited to one per day. Patients should also be closely monitored for at least one hour after meals and snacks for purging. They should have daily weights, vital signs, and lab draw for electrolytes.

Bulimia nervosa

For many years bulimia nervosa and anorexia nervosa were considered to be the same eating disorder. However, bulimia has many different characteristics and is an entirely different type of disorder. This type of eating disorder is actually more common than anorexia and outcomes are usually better with lower mortality rates. The usual age of onset is a little older than anorexia and is between the ages of 15 to 18 years. It is more common in females; however, symptoms are the same in both sexes. Signs and symptoms of bulimia are not as obvious and many times go unnoticed by friends and family. These individuals will binge eat and purge in secret and can be thin, normal weight, or overweight.

Associated psychological findings
Many of the patients seeking help for eating disorders will often have other comorbid psychiatric disorders. They commonly have major depression, dysthymia, anxiety disorders, and substance abuse problems. The presence of obsessive-compulsive disorder, post traumatic stress disorder, and mood disorders are also commonly found in this patient population. Individuals with personality disorders are also more likely to have bulimia nervosa than the general population. Symptoms can include perfectionism, rigidity, ritualism, and increased risk avoidance and self control. Many patients report feelings of helplessness, guilt, shame, low-self esteem, and difficulty identifying feelings or managing intense emotions.

Physical and laboratory findings
Many of the physical and laboratory findings associated with bulimia nervosa are due to poor nutrition and self-induced vomiting habits. Physical symptoms can include loss of dental enamel or increased dental caries, chipped teeth, scars on dorsum of hand, cardiac and skeletal muscle myopathies, esophageal tears with associated bleeding, amenorrhea or irregular menstrual cycles, and decreased normal GI functioning due to overuse of laxatives. Some of the associated laboratory findings include fluid and electrolyte imbalances with increased BUN and hypokalemia, metabolic alkalosis or acidosis, and elevated amylase levels.

Diagnostic characteristics
There are two different types of bulimia nervosa and they include the purging type and restrictive type. Patients with restrictive type are similar in symptoms to anorexia; however, after they restrict their eating for a period of time, they will then binge eat and purge. This will become a

cycle of behavior for these individuals. Key diagnostic criteria for bulimia includes repetitive cycles of binge eating and use of inappropriate behaviors to prevent weight gain, such as induced vomiting; overuse of laxatives, diuretics or enemas; excessive exercise; or fasting. With bulimia, the individual will have binge eating along with inappropriate behaviors to prevent weight gain at least two times a week for at least 3 months and is highly influenced by body weight and shape when describing self. With the purging type, the individual will frequently utilize self-induced vomiting, laxatives, or diuretics in compensation for binge eating. In the nonpurging type, they will frequently fast, exercise excessively, and may or may not use laxatives and diuretics.

Binge eating disorder and night eating syndrome

Binge eating disorder and night eating syndrome also are included under the umbrella of eating disorders. In binge eating disorder, the person binge eats large quantities of food; however, they do not attempt any compensatory activities to prevent weight gain. This particular disorder only affects a small percentage of the population; however, the incidence of this disorder is approximately 20-40% in obese individuals seeking treatment for their obesity. With night eating syndrome, the individuals have morning time anorexia, depression symptoms in the evening, and problems with insomnia. These individuals usually awaken twice during the night and eat during this time.

Dementia

Dementia is a loss of cognition that leads to impaired functioning of an individual's normal activities. It is usually irreversible and slow in onset. These individuals will maintain a normal level of consciousness and are usually able to concentrate on a single task for a long period of time. The most common type of dementia is Alzheimer's dementia. Impairment of short-term memory is often the first noticeable symptom. Later in the disease process, agnosia, apraxia, and aphasia may also occur along with many personality changes. Depression, disordered reasoning, disorientation, confabulation, and amnesia may also be associated with this type of dementia.

Other types of dementia include vascular dementia, Lewy body dementia, HIV related dementia, and frontal-temporal dementia. There are also less common dementia types that are related to specific disease processes such as Parkinson's, Huntington's, neurosyphilis, and Creutzfeldt-Jacob disease. Dementia can also be related to head trauma, a genetic predisposition, substance abuse, or exposure to certain toxins. Distinguishing between different types or causes is often impossible with definitive diagnosis not occurring until a postmortem exam in completed. Vascular dementia is the second most common type of dementia with both embolic and hemorrhagic CVA, transient ischemic attacks (TIAs), cerebral atrophy, and atherosclerosis being commonly found.

<u>Pathophysiology of Alzheimer's dementia</u>
The exact cause of Alzheimer's dementia has not yet been identified. It is known that neurons are lost and this leads to a disruption of normal neurotransmission and decreased levels of acetylcholine leading to a decline in cholinergic activity. Characteristic neuritic plaques and neurofibrillary tangles are often found. Neuritic plaques are composed of a buildup of cellular material and a protein called beta-amyloid around the neurons. This plaque buildup is highest in the occipital and temporal lobes of the brain. These plaques are associated with symptoms such as aphasia and visuospatial abnormalities. Neurofibrillary tangles occur when nerve fibers surrounding the hippocampus become entangled causing improper transmission of information and eventually result in cell death. These tangles are associated with memory loss and many of the psychiatric symptoms.

<u>Diagnostic criteria for Alzheimer's dementia</u>
The key diagnostic characteristics for diagnosis of Alzheimer's dementia include the following:
- Development of several cognitive deficits.
- Memory impairment plus at least one of the following disturbances: aphasia, apraxia, agnosia, or disturbed executive functioning.
- Significant decline in social and occupational functioning from previous levels as a result of cognitive impairment.
- Causes of cognitive deficits not related to any other medical disease process or substance abuse induced. No better explained by another Axis I disorder.
- Occurs apart from an episode of delirium.

Delirium

Delirium is an acute transient state in which there is impairment in consciousness and altered cognition. This confusional state is most commonly seen in the very old or very young and is often brought on by a wide variety of physiological causes, such as fever, infection, fluid and electrolyte imbalances, or hypoxia. It can also be medication induced or occur due to medication or substance withdrawal. Common symptoms can include change in level of consciousness, inability to focus, disorientation, memory disturbances, rambling speech, inability to carry on a normal conversation, or inability to recognize familiar objects. The onset of delirium is abrupt and symptoms develop over a short time frame and may fluctuate during different times of the day. It is usually reversible if the cause is identified early and treated.

In children, delirium if often the result of fever or anticholinergic medications. In the elderly, delirium can be life-threatening and is often the result of medications. These medications may include anticholinergics, salicylates, steroids, sedatives, insulin, cardiac glycosides, antipsychotics, or anticonvulsants. Other causes can include infection; surgery; hypoxia; endocrine dysfunctions; electrolyte abnormalities; cardiovascular disease; or disease processes of the lung, kidney, or liver. An imbalance of neurotransmitters may play an important role in the development of delirium. An imbalance in dopamine, norepinephrine, or acetylcholine can cause many alterations in the brain that can lead to delirium. A reciprocal relationship involving Dopamine seems to occur. Dopamine levels increase and reuptake decreases. This can cause an increase in excitation. Alzheimer's patients are highly susceptible to delirium due to impaired cholinergic transmission associated with this disease.

Metabolic disorders and cerebral functioning

Many metabolic disorders can cause impairment in cognition. The longer the metabolic disturbance exists, the more likely there is to be a decline in an individual's mental status. Hypoxia, endocrine disease (hypo or hyper), neoplastic tumors, hypothalamic disease, and nutritional deficits can all play a role. Hypoxia can result from decreased respiratory or cardiac functioning, dehydration, or decreased hemoglobin and hematocrit (H&H). A decrease in H&H can be from acute GI bleeding or from iron, folic acid, or B12 deficiency. Mental status changes due to hypoxia occur because of a decrease in available oxygen to the brain. Endocrine disorders, such as hyper or hypothyroidism, hypoglycemia, or adrenal disease can lead to a deterioration or change in mental status. Hypothalamic disease can result in an inability to control body temperature. Malnutrition is commonly seen in individuals with eating disorders or alcohol abuse, the elderly, low income, or homeless populations.

Pathophysiology of addiction

Genetic, social, and personality factors may all play a role in the development of addictive tendencies. However, the main factor of the development of substance addiction is the pharmacological activation of the reward system located in the central nervous system (CNS). This reward systems pathway involves dopaminergic neurons. Dopamine is found in the CNS and is one of many neurotransmitters that play a role in an individual's mood. The mesolimbic pathway seems to play a primary role in the reward and motivational process involved with addiction. This pathway begins in the ventral tegmental area of the brain (VTA) and then moves forward into the nucleus accumbens located in the middle forebrain bundle (MFB). Some drugs enhance mesolimbic dopamine activity, therefore producing very potent effects on mood and behavior.

Substance abuse disorders

Substance abuse disorders are behaviors related to taking an abusive drug such as alcohol, amphetamines, marijuana, cocaine, hallucinogens, sedatives, or other unidentified substances. This group of disorders is classified into four different categories that include substance dependence, substance abuse, substance intoxication, and substance withdrawal. The United States has one of the highest rates of substance abuse when compared to other countries. It is a chronic disease process with many relapses. It is a huge cost to the US, with substance abusers utilizing a large amount of health care dollars. These individual will have long term serious medical sequela associated with abuse, along with frequent hospitalizations and emergency department visits.

Effects of alcohol abuse

Alcohol is a CNS depressant, or sedative-hypnotic, which depresses tissues within the brain. These drugs decrease anxiety and/or induce sleep. Even though alcohol is a sedative, it also causes a sense of euphoria. Its effects also include decreased inhibitions, relaxation, impaired coordination, slurred speech, and nausea. In cases of toxicity and overdose it can cause respiratory depression leading to respiratory or cardiac arrest. Withdrawal symptoms can include shaking, seizures, hyperthermia, tachycardia, hypertension, and delirium. Long term complications can affect all body systems and lead to death.

Abuse of amphetamines and cocaine

Amphetamines and cocaine are both classified as CNS stimulants. They can both be taken orally or injected. Cocaine can also be smoked or used topically. These drugs cause a sudden sensation of euphoria, energy, wakefulness, diminished appetite, and insomnia. They can also cause paranoia, aggressiveness, dilated pupils, shaking, hyperactivity, pressured speech, constipation, dry mouth, tachycardia, and chest pain. An overdose can lead to sudden cardiac death or myocardial infarction due to coronary artery spasm, cardiac dysrhythmias, hyper or hypotension, respiratory depression or arrest, seizures, psychosis, dyskinesias, dystonias, coma, or death. Withdrawal symptoms can include feelings of depression and fatigue with suicidal ideations, agitation, insomnia, anxiety, nightmares, and increased appetite. These drugs are often alternated with depressants and can result in malnutrition or a schizophrenia-like syndrome.

Abuse of barbiturates and benzodiazepines

Barbiturates and benzodiazepines are classified as CNS depressants or sedative-hypnotics. These drugs can be taken orally or injected. Their effects include depression of the major brain functions such as mood, cognition, memory, insight, or judgment and can cause feelings of euphoria and emotional lability. They can also lead to sedation and decreased sexual desire. Overdose can lead to unresponsiveness, coma, respiratory, and cardiac arrest. Withdrawal symptoms can include anxiety and agitation, hypertension, tachycardia, diaphoresis, increased temperature, excitability, insomnia, seizures, delirium, or hallucinations. Long term complications can include those acquired from shared needle use as well as medical conditions associated with other dependencies.

Physiologic response involved with opiates

Opiates are powerful pain relievers and many are utilized medically for pain control. Examples of opiates include heroine, morphine, meperidine, codeine, and methadone. There are three types of opiate related drugs: agonists that increase the central nervous system effects, antagonists that block these effects, and mixed agonist-antagonists. Opiates act by elevating the production of dopamine by increasing the neuronal firing rate of dopamine producing cells. The opiate abuser's mood is elevated resulting in a sense of euphoria brought on by the increased dopamine activity. Opiate receptors are located throughout the brain and body and are activated by endorphins.

Physiologic response involved with stimulants

Stimulants such as cocaine and amphetamines increase levels of dopamine, serotonin, and norepinephrine in the synapse. However, the mechanisms between the two differ somewhat. Cocaine inhibits the monoamine reuptake mechanism. The inhibition of reuptake increases dopamine levels and leads to a rewarding sense of euphoria. Cocaine's effect is usually short lived and the abuser will repeat the abuse to achieve the desired effect. Amphetamines both increase the release of norepinephrine and dopamine and also inhibit their reuptake.

Cannabis abuse

Cannabis includes hashish; THC; and marijuana, also known as grass, dope, joint, weed, or J. They can be used by smoking or taken orally. These drugs alter the user's state of awareness and can cause euphoria or dysphoria, sleepiness, heightened color and sound perceptions, red eyes, decreased inhibitions, dry mouth, increased appetite, or tingling sensations. Overdose can lead to tachycardia, disorientation, or toxic psychosis. There are usually no associated withdrawal symptoms; however, users can become irritable and may have insomnia for a few days. No long term medication complications usually occur, however the individual may experience an inability to concentrate and experience some memory disturbances.

Opiate abuse

Opiates include heroine, morphine, meperidine, codeine, opium, and methadone. All of the drugs can be given orally except meperidine, which can only be given by injection. Opium can also be smoked. Heroine, morphine, codeine, and meperidine can also be given by injection. These drugs cause a sense of euphoria, relaxation, pain relief, sedation, decreased sexual desire, impaired judgment, constricted pupils, nausea, slurred speech, and memory and concentration impairment. Overdose can lead to unresponsiveness, coma, or respiratory and cardiovascular depression leading to arrest and death. Withdrawal symptoms include watery eyes, runny nose, yawning, dilated pupils, goose bumps, diaphoresis, GI upset, insomnia, anorexia, flushing, hypertension, paresthesias, headaches, and fatigue. Chronic use can lead to malnutrition and dehydration along with medical problems caused by use of dirty needles.

PCP abuse

Phencyclidine (PCP) can be taken orally or smoked to achieve the desired effects. This drug causes the user to feel as if they are superhuman. They have enhanced strength and endurance and will often experience intense rage. They may become agitated and hyperactive, acting out violently, or they may become catatonic and withdrawn or move back and forth between the two states. They may also have an increased pain threshold and stimulation of the cardiovascular and respiratory systems. In overdose, they may experience hallucinations, paranoia, psychosis, adrenergic crisis, cardiac arrest, stroke, malignant hyperthermia, seizures, or death. There are usually no associated withdrawal side effects. Long term problems can include mild flashbacks or organic brain syndromes with psychosis lasting up to 6 months after drug use was discontinued. These individuals commonly have frequent police arrests.

Abuse of hallucinogens

Hallucinogens include LSD; DMT; mescaline; and MDMA, also known as ecstasy. These drugs can be taken orally or smoked. Effects can include distorted or sharpened visual and hearing perceptions, hallucinations, distortions of space and time, depersonalization, mystical experiences, mood lability, euphoria or dysphoria, altered body image, bizarre behaviors, confusion, impaired judgment and memory, dilated pupils, diaphoresis, palpitations, or panic reactions. Overdose symptoms can include paranoia, seizures, hyperthermia, hallucinations, or death. There are usually no withdrawal side effects and long term problems may include flashbacks that may last for many months or the user may develop a chronic state of psychosis.

Abuse of inhalants

Abuse of inhalants can include use of glue, aerosol sprays, paint thinners, or lighter fluid. Using inhalants can cause the user to feel a sense of euphoria and giddiness. It can also cause impaired judgment, apathy, and assaultive behaviors. Overdose of these drugs causes CNS depression, dizziness, slurred speech, nystagmus, unsteady gait, dysarthria, shaking, depressed reflexes, and decreased appetite. In overdose, these drugs can lead to coma, seizures, respiratory or cardiac arrest, and death. Withdrawal symptoms are very similar to those seen with alcohol withdrawal; however, they are usually milder. Long-term use can lead to liver and kidney disease, blood disorders, interstitial lung disease, CNS damage, or permanent cognitive impairment that could require placement in a long term care facility.

Family

A family consists of a group of people that are connected by marriage, blood relationship, or emotionally. There are many different variations when referring to the concept of family. The nuclear family is one in which two or more people are related by blood, marriage, or adoption. This type of family is typically parents and their children. The extended family is one in which several nuclear families related by blood or marriage function as one group. A household consists of an individual or group of people residing together under one roof. The nurse will often interact with families on many different levels. This may involve meeting the family once during the patient's treatment or establishing a long-term relationship with the family over the course of a chronically ill psychiatric patient's treatment.

Functional family

A functional family will be able to change roles, responsibilities, and interactions during a stressful event. This type of family can experience nonfunctional behaviors if placed in an acute stressful event; however, they should be able to reestablish their family balance over a period of time. The functional family will have the ability to deal with conflict and change in order to deal with negative situations without causing long-term dysfunction or dissolution of the family. They will have completed vital life cycle tasks, keep emotional contact between family members and across generations, over-closeness is avoided, and distance is used to resolve issues. When two members of the family have a conflict, they are expected to resolve this conflict between themselves and there is open communication between all family members. Children of a functional family are expected to achieve age appropriate functioning and are given age appropriate privileges.

Cultural and ethnic differences within the family

Different cultural and ethnic backgrounds can affect the definition of family. They may have different beliefs about the functions of family members. Conflict may be resolved differently within families, and adaptive and maladaptive responses may vary. Outside events may be viewed differently and interventions within the family may differ between cultural groups. Many times African American and Latino families often look to other family members instead of health care professionals for support early in the problem. These families also have higher rates of attrition and termination of family therapy than Caucasian families.

Effects of mental illness on the family

Families with a member that has a chronic mental illness will provide several functions that those without mentally ill members may not need. These functions can include providing support and information for care and treatment options. They will also monitor the services provided the family member and address concerns with these services. Many times the family is the biggest advocate for additional availability of services for mental health patients. There can often be disagreements between the health care providers and the family members concerning the dependence of the patient within the family. Parents can often be viewed as overprotective when attempting to encourage patient independence and self-reliant functioning. They will need support and reassurance if the individual leaves home. On the other hand, many parents will provide for their child for as long as they live. Once the primary care provider dies, the patient may be left with no one to care for them and they may experience traumatic disruptions.

Family life cycle

The family life cycle is a process in which the family undergoes changes to allow for the introduction of new family members, exiting of existing family members, and the development of present family members in a positive functional manner. This cycle is described in stages and includes times of transition. Many times stress and dysfunction can occur during these times of transition and the family may seek assistance to be able to successfully navigate this period of time. The stages of the family life cycle include leaving home as a young adult, joining of families though marriage or establishment of an emotional relationship, having young children, having adolescent children, launching young adult children and moving forward, and finally the family later in life.

Family violence

Family violence can include physical, emotional, sexual, or verbal behaviors that occur between members of the same family or others living within the home. This behavior can include both abuse and neglect and involve the elderly, spouses, and children. Family violence is often kept a secret and may be the main issue with many family problems. Many times, actions that would be considered unacceptable to strangers or friends are often the norm between family members. Violence and abuse occur due to the unique interactions between the family members based upon personality differences, situational variations, and sociocultural influences.

Violent families will often share many of the same characteristics. Many times the abusive family member will have suffered abuse from their family while growing up. This type of abuse is multigenerational transmission and is a cycle of violence. These abusers have learned to believe that violent behavior is a way to solve problems. Violent families are also usually socially isolated so that others such as friends, teachers, neighbors or law enforcement officials do not become aware that the abuse is occurring. The abuser will also use and abuse power to control the victim. They may be considered a person of authority, such as a parent would be to a child. Power is a very important factor with abuse of an intimate partner. The abuser is often very controlling of their partner and will attempt to dominate every aspect of their life. Another commonality among abusers is substance abuse; however, one is not dependent upon the other. Many times the use of alcohol or drugs may escalate violent behaviors by decreasing inhibitions.

Sexuality

Sexuality is an integral part of each individual's personality and refers to all aspects of being a sexual human. It is more than just the act of physical intercourse. A person's sexuality is often apparent in everything they do, their appearance, and how they interact with other people. There are four main aspects of sexuality and they include the following: genetic identity or chromosomal gender, gender identification or how they perceive themselves with regards to male or female, gender role or the attributes of their cultural role, and sexual orientation or the gender to which one is attracted. By assessing and attempting to conceptualize a person's sexuality, the health care provider can gain a broader understanding of the patient's beliefs and will be able to provide a more holistic approach to providing care.

Effects of medications
There are many different types of medications that can lead to sexual dysfunction. Medications such as antihypertensives, anticholinergics, neuroleptics, antiseizure, benzodiazepines, antipsychotics, and SSRIs are all examples of medication types that can cause sexual dysfunction. With anticholinergics and antiseizure medications, the side effects can include a decreased libido or orgasmic disorders in both men and women. SSRIs can cause a disruption in any phase of the sexual response. Women commonly complain of anorgasmia or delayed orgasm. Men also complain of anorgasmia plus additional problems with ejaculation. Many of these side effects lead to patient noncompliance and they will stop taking their medications in order to avoid these side effects. Many times the medication or dosage can be changed to help combat these side effects.

Psychiatric illness and sexuality
Many times psychiatric illness can affect a person's sexuality. Mental illness, such as depression, can often decrease the patient's sexual desire, but then the manic patient will often become hypersexual. Bipolar patients can experience a lack of sexual inhibition and may have many sexual affairs or act very seductively or overtly sexual. Psychotic patients may experience hallucinations or delusions of a sexual nature, and the schizophrenic patient may exhibit inappropriate sexual behaviors such as masturbation in public. Long term care facilities will need to keep their residents safe from sexually transmitted diseases, unwanted pregnancies, and unwanted sexual advances or assaults from others.

Neurologic and psychiatric complications of HIV

Many of the individuals infected with HIV will have both neurologic and psychological complications that occur as a result of the disease process. Many times neurologic complications occur as a result of brain infections, such as meningitis or encephalitis, which lead to cognitive and motor function abnormalities. This syndrome is called the HIV-1-associated cognitive-motor complex. HIV is thought to cause the brain to release high levels of neurotoxins and excitatory amino acids, which ultimately cause cell death. Many of these patients will also develop AIDS dementia, which leads to alterations in orientation and personality. In the later stages the patient will often develop delirium, dementia, or organic mood disorder. Many of these patients will also suffer from major depression after diagnosis.

Psychological impact of pain

Pain affects both the physical and psychological well being of the individual. It encompasses both a sensory and emotional response. A patient will cope with pain through many different behavioral responses. Acute pain is associated with an immediate occurring problem and is usually resolved in a few months or less. Fear, expectations, coping abilities, or cultural influences can all affect a patient's response to pain. A change in normal sleep patterns, anorexia, anxiety, or agitation can occur. Chronic pain is pain that lasts longer than six months. Chronic pain can lead to neurochemical abnormalities and depression. A complete assessment and evaluation of the pain should be performed and documented. Appropriate diagnosis and treatment plan should be in place to assist with successful treatment of pain.

Anger, aggression, and violence

Both violence and aggressive behaviors are commonly seen in the psychiatric and mental health population. Violence is a physical act perpetrated against an inanimate object, animal, or other person with the intent to cause harm. This action is often the result of anger, frustration, or fear and often occurs because the perpetrator believes that they are threatened or that their opinion is right and the victim is wrong. This act can often result in death or severe injury. Aggression is the communication of a threat or intended act of violence and will often occur before the act of violence. This communication can occur verbally or nonverbally. Gestures, increased volume of voice, invasion of personal space, or prolonged eye contact can all be examples of nonverbal aggression.

Associated areas of the brain

The three main areas of the brain associated with altered aggression, anger, and violence include the limbic system, frontal lobes, and the hypothalamus. The limbic system is involved with the processing of information, memory, and emotions. The area known as the amygdale is particularly involved in the expression of rage and fear. Alterations in this system may result in altered levels of anger and violence. The frontal lobes are involved with reasoning and intentional behaviors. Trauma to this area of the brain can lead to personality changes, angry emotional outbursts, or impaired decision making abilities. The hypothalamus is involved with the body's stress response system. This area of the brain sends messages to the pituitary gland to raise steroid levels within the body in response to stress. Malfunctions of the hypothalamus can lead to overstimulation and abnormally elevated levels of steroids.

<u>Biologic etiologies</u>
Biologic etiologies associated with increased anger, aggression, and violence have been associated with the functioning of certain areas of the brain. There are three main areas that may be related: the limbic system, frontal lobes, and the hypothalamus. Abnormal neurotransmitters, such as low serotonin levels, are also associated with altered expressions of anger and violence. Other biologic influences that may influence a person's aggressive behaviors can include malnutrition, developmental deficits, tumors, trauma, or degenerative processes of the brain. These biological factors can interact with other influences, such as a family history of violence, drug or alcohol abuse, schizophrenia, or noncompliance with medication regimes, to produce increased anger responses.

<u>Psychological causes</u>
Psychological aspects of increased anger, aggression, and violence can be associated with uncontrollable instinctual urges or as a result of the person's particular life experiences. Exposure to violence, altered mother/child bonding, altered socialization skills, or reinforcement of aggressive behavior by achievement of a goal can all lead to increased utilization of aggression and violence. Overexposure to violence through the media, entertainment, or their immediate environment can possibly lead to a desensitization of aggression and violence and lead to maladaptive behavioral responses.

Nursing diagnosis

The nursing diagnosis is created based upon a clinical judgment about an individual or group. A problem, need, or vulnerability associated with the individual or group is identified along with any associated risk factors. Then nursing interventions or management is created to assist with the identified actual or potential problem. This diagnosis is based upon the information gathered during the nursing assessment. The diagnosis includes a concise statement, key characteristics, and any related factors. The creation of a diagnosis and implementation of the treatment plan is performed by the nurse. Many of these diagnoses are taken from the NANDA-approved list of nursing diagnosis.

Nursing process

The nursing process is individualized to each and every patient. It includes a systematic approach at solving actual problems or preventing potential problems. It builds on the nurse-patient relationship and moves towards the goal of the patient developing a new set of adaptive skills. Psychiatric patients can present complex issues that often present less definitively than physical medical disease processes. Many of the symptoms overlap or are vaguely described by the patient. Often times the patient doesn't even know exactly what they are experiencing. They can be under stress or anxiety and may be experiencing many symptoms at once. The nurse should empower the patient to participate in their care decisions and goal setting. This increases self-esteem and provides the patient with a sense of choice.

Patient outcomes

Patient outcomes are a description of the patient's response to nursing interventions. The outcome statement describes what is expected and is stated in exact measurable terms. Nursing diagnosis and interventions are linked to the outcome statement. This association allows for the documentation and measurement of the effectiveness of the nursing intervention over time. Outcomes can be the actual patient response or the status of a diagnosis. Through evaluation of patient outcomes, measurable evidence is created on which nursing practice can be based. The overall goal of outcome measurement is to provide quality patient care.

Evaluation

The main purpose of evaluating patient outcomes is to assure the delivery of quality care. Patient outcome measures drive the process of quality improvement. These outcomes provide a framework for an expected patient response based on current medical knowledge. By monitoring and documenting patient outcomes, negative trends or variations can be identified and then measures put in place to decrease these trends. Through identification of negative variables, nursing interventions can be added or removed to positively affect patient outcomes. Patients can also utilize outcome measurements to achieve feelings of success when they attain a specific outcome.

Documentation

Psychiatric nurses are not only responsible for creating nursing diagnoses and interventions and evaluating outcomes, but they are also responsible for their proper documentation. This documentation is utilized to determine the success of treatment as well as its cost effectiveness. These outcomes are measured against many different things that may affect the patient while being treated, such as physical illness, coping abilities, functional status, and overall patient and family satisfaction. This data collection can be utilized to determine program development, budgets, and staffing related issues. The main outcomes to be evaluated include clinical, satisfaction, functional, and financial outcomes.

Crisis

A crisis occurs when a person is faced with a highly stressful event and their usual problem solving and coping skills fail to be effective in resolving the situation. This event usually leads to increased levels of anxiety and can bring about a physical and psychological response. The problem is usually an acute event that can be identified. It may have occurred a few weeks or even months before or immediately prior to the crisis and can be an actual event or a potential event. The crisis state usually lasts less than six weeks with the individual then becoming able to utilize problem solving skills to cope effectively. A person in crisis does not always have a mental disorder. However, during the acute crisis their social functioning and decision making abilities may be impaired.

There are basically two different types of crises. These types include developmental or maturational crisis and situational crisis. A developmental crisis can occur during maturation when an individual must take on a new life role. This crisis can be a normal part of the developmental process. A youth may need to face crisis and resolve this crisis to be able to move on to the next developmental stage. This may occur during the process of moving from adolescence to adulthood. Examples of situations that could lead to this type of crisis include graduating from school, going away to college, or moving out on their own. These situations would cause the individual to face a maturing event that requires the development of new coping skills.

The second type of crisis is the situational crisis. This type of crisis can occur at any time in life. There is usually an event or problem that occurs, which leads to a disruption in normal psychological functioning. These types of events are often unplanned and can occur with or without warning. Some examples that may lead to a situational crisis include the death of a loved one, divorce, unplanned or unwanted pregnancy, onset or change in a physical disease process, job loss, or being the victim of a violent act. Events that affect an entire community can also cause individual and community situation crisis. Terrorist attacks or weather related disasters are examples of events that can affect an entire community.

Individualization of the patient plan of care

The individualization of the patient plan of care is essential to its success. Each patient presents with their own set of problems or vulnerabilities. Treatment plans and outcomes should reflect each specific patient. The nurse should also realize that each patient presents with their own goals in mind and these should be evaluated and documented. Educational, social, and cultural influences will greatly affect the plan of care. Patient specific learning preferences and needs should be well documented so that other health care providers can be aware of their individual wants and needs.

Continuum of care

The continuum of care can move from inpatient treatments to various outpatient treatments and support systems. This allows for varying levels of intensity throughout the patient treatment program. It allows for treatment to be coordinated in many different environmental settings, care levels, by different health care providers, and by a variety of different services. This continuum of care occurs over a long period of time and includes the involvement of many different services. Its purpose is to meet the comprehensive needs of the patient through the coordination of interdisciplinary care and services.

The continuum of care occurs throughout the course of treatment for the individual patient. This may begin with acute crisis intervention and stabilization in the hospital setting and may then move to partial hospitalization allowing for the patient to leave for periods of time or go home at night. Residential services are included in this continuum and may provide a place for patients to stay at any time during the day or night. Services provided here can include medical treatments, nursing care, psychosocial care, vocational training, or recreational diversion. Respite care can provide short-term relief housing and care for psychiatric patients living at home with their family. Outpatient treatment programs as well as supportive employment programs also participate in the provision of the continuum of care.

Stages of grief

The death of a loved one can be a very common reason for someone to experience a crisis. The person must move through the grief to resolve the crisis. The first stage of grief is shock and the person will often experience feelings of denial. Physical symptoms can include shortness of air, sensations of choking, or feeling faint. During this time the individual may feel isolated. The second stage of grief includes acute mourning. This starts when the person begins to believe that the loss is real. There are usually three phases that include intense feelings, social withdrawal, and then identification with the person that has been lost. The phase of intense feelings includes symptoms of intense pain. The individual may often become tearful and cry. In the phase of social withdrawal, the individual avoids social and emotional contact with others. In the phase of identification with the person they have lost, the individual becomes engulfed with thoughts of the deceased.

In some instances the stages of grief can take years for the individual to complete. The final stage of grief is the resolution phase. This is when the loss is finally accepted and the person begins to feel as though they may be able to return to their normal life functions. They may begin to be able to think and talk about the deceased without experiencing the intense pain associated with acute mourning. They come to a realization that they have been grieving and are ready to look to the future and rejoin social groups and accept the friendship of others.

Delayed grief reaction

A delayed grief reaction may occur when an event triggers the grief process that was not completed at the time of the death. The person is experiencing a dysfunctional grieving process. Symptoms of a delayed grief reaction can include anger and hostility, feelings of emptiness or numbness lasting for a long period of time, inability to weep or experience emotions of grief, continued use of the present tense instead of the past tense when referring to the deceased, continued dreaming about the loss, continuing to keep personal belongings, or inability to visit the grave site of the deceased. Many times the individual will hold onto an object in place of the loved one and place living memories into this object.

Discharge planning

Discharge planning starts with the admission assessment. The goal for any inpatient admission is to successfully guide the patient through their crisis and be discharged from the facility. After discharge, the patient will need to be referred or transferred for ongoing care. With the admission of the patient, the nurse will need to begin to evaluate their discharge situation and any needs. This allows for the follow-up plan to begin to be formed. The patient should have access to the resources they will need to continue to function successfully as an outpatient. Discharge planning involves communication between several different resources to provide continuity of care and to decrease the potential for readmission to the inpatient facility. The patient and family should be included in the decision making process and given information regarding support services.

Learning

Hands-on and verbal styles
Every person has a very individualized way of learning and processing information. Upon admission a patient should be evaluated for their preferred method of learning. This information allows the health care providers to provide patient education in a manner that is best suited to each patient. Successful patient education is a vital part of the patient's recovery and continued successful coping and functioning throughout their life. Learning styles can include auditory, visual, hands-on, or verbal. A person that learns best through tactile or hands-on education prefers to receive the information through touch and doing. They may have difficulty sitting for long periods of time and prefer to be actively involved in the education process. A verbal learner often thinks in words instead of pictures. They are often great speakers and listeners. They have the ability to understand the meanings of words and are great at remembering information.

Auditory and visual styles
People learn in many different ways. Most people favor a particular type of learning style that allows them to process the information in the best way possible. Each patient should be evaluated to determine their preferred learning style. Learning styles can include auditory, visual, hands-on, and verbal. A person that learns best through auditory models can process information best through the act of listening. They prefer to receive information through discussions, lectures, and by talking through and listening to information given by others. Visual learners process information best through the use of pictures, videos, written information, or diagrams. Many times these learners need to see the body language and gestures of the person teaching.

Barriers

Many times psychiatric patients may have many different barriers to learning that can impact patient education. Upon admission to an inpatient facility, many patients may be in crisis and unable to take in the simples instructions. The patient may need further education on the same information after they have moved through their crisis stage. Other barriers can include visual, hearing, physical, or cognitive impairments. Patients should be individually evaluated for their preferred method of receiving information. Ability to read or a patient's educational level will also affect which type of information is best suited for that specific patient. Cultural and language barriers should also be evaluated and considered when providing patient and family education.

Implementation and Evaluation of Comprehensive Plan of Care

Psychopharmacology

Most psychiatric patients receive some sort of psychopharmacology treatment. With increased public education on many mental health disorders, pharmacological treatments are on the rise. Psychiatric medications mainly affect the central nervous system. More specifically, these medications affect actions at the cellular and synaptic level. It is very important that nurses understand exactly how these medications will affect their patients. Different symptoms will require the use of different medications. Specific drugs will act in specific ways. The nurse will need to understand how to administer these medications, their actions, and potential side effects. Many times drug therapy is used in conjunction with other therapies such as counseling or behavior modification.

Nurse's role

The role of the nurse in psychopharmacology is very important. The nurse must understand each medication and what effects it may have on the patient. Documentation of a complete patient assessment is vital to the evaluation process of any medication. An assessment should be performed before initiation of treatment to determine the patient's baseline. An assessment should also be performed during treatment to evaluate for any change in symptoms or presence of side effects. The nurse also has an important role in patient education. Many psychiatric medications can have extreme side effects that the patient's themselves should monitor. Education should also include, benefits, dosage, frequency, lifestyle effects, and whom to contact for any problems.

Role of a receptor site

Most medications are developed for use by a specific receptor site within the body. Receptors are located on the cellular membrane and act to allow molecules to affect the action of the cell. Naturally occurring neurotransmitters or medications acting as neurotransmitters modify the body's receptor site by bonding with them. A drug that acts as an agonist produces the same effects as the neurotransmitter and stimulates this receptor. When a drug acts as an antagonist, it blocks the receptor site, therefore inhibiting the action of the cell by other agonists.

Metabolism of psychiatric medications

Many of the mediations used to treat mental illness are taken orally. These medications are absorbed by the gastrointestinal (GI) tract and then move on to the liver for metabolism. The liver alters much of the medication causing it to be unavailable for use by the body. More specifically, many of these medications are metabolized by a specific enzyme in the liver called CYP 450. Certain medications are greatly affected by the first-pass effect. The first pass effect is when an organ in the body acts to greatly reduce the effectiveness of the drug by decreasing the drugs availability for systemic circulation. Drug levels in the body are determined by the body's ability to metabolize these medications.

Drug availability within the body

There are many factors that may affect drug availability within the body. The route that a mediation is given can determine systemic availability of that medication. The availability of a drug given orally can be reduced by a high first pass effect or diminished absorption of the drug in the GI tract due to increased or decreased motility or altered nutritional status. Conversely, medications that are given by IV or IM often have higher systemic availability because they are not subject to the same type of absorption or metabolism effects seen with oral medications. Often times the same medication is given at greatly reduced dosages when given by IV or IM when compared to the oral dosage.

Potency and efficacy of medication

The potency and efficacy of a medication helps to guide health care providers with medication choices. The potency of a medication is determined by how much drug produces the desired effect and is an important consideration when comparing medications. One medication may produce the same response as another but utilizes less medication to achieve it. This would make the drug more potent than the other. The efficacy of a drug is its ability to elicit a physiologic response from the receptor. A medication with increased efficacy will produce a greater response than one with low efficacy. A medication may be very potent but have low efficacy.

Selectivity, affinity, and intrinsic activity of medications

A medication has the ability to bond with a particular receptor site due to its selectivity, affinity, or intrinsic activity. Selectivity refers to the medications ability to bond only with specific receptors. It selects the target receptor type from all others. It will not interact with unwanted cells of other organs or tissues and can help reduce certain side effects. Affinity describes the intensity of the attraction between the medication and its receptor site. If the drug has a high affinity, its effects will last longer and it is less likely that another drug will knock it off of its receptor site. The intrinsic activity of a drug describes its ability to produce the desired physiologic response. An example of a drug that would not produce an intrinsic response is an antagonist. It bonds selectively and may have strong affinity but does not act to produce a physiologic response. It acts to block one.

Phases of pharmacological treatment

There are four main phases of pharmacological treatment. These include initiation, stabilization, maintenance, and discontinuation. The nurse is involved in all phases of this treatment process and patient assessment during the phases is vital. It must be determined if the patient is actually taking the medication as it was prescribed and if the desired effect is achieved. Careful assessment and documentation will provide insight into which phase the patient is in and if they are progressing as expected. Alterations of the medication can be made based upon the patient's response during any of these phases.

Initiation phase
The initiation phase involves a complete assessment and patient history. A complete picture of the patient must be obtained to assist in determining which medication should be utilized. Lab work such as blood chemistry; complete blood count; and liver, kidney, and thyroid function tests should be obtained. Certain medication dosages may need to be adjusted based on these results. The

presence of any physical condition should also be ruled out as a cause of symptoms. The inpatient should be closely monitored with the first dose of any medication for adverse reactions.

Stabilization phase

The stabilization phase is the time in which the proper dosage of medication is determined. There may need to be increases or decreases in dosage to achieve the desired response with minimal side effects. There should be an ongoing assessment process. This should include physical and psychological assessments along with re-evaluation of certain lab values or drug levels. The patient should be closely monitored for any unwanted side effects of adverse reactions such as abnormal muscle movements or elevated blood pressure or temperature. The initial medication chosen may not produce the desired response and it may require the addition of another medication or be discontinued altogether. The patient should be closely monitored for any drug interactions.

Maintenance phase

During the maintenance phase a medication is utilized to prevent reoccurrence of the unwanted symptoms. Occasionally, these symptoms may reappear even though the medication is continued. This can occur because of a change in metabolism caused by the medication, development of tolerance, physical illness, stress, or use of additional prescription or over the counter medications. Some side effects may not be evident until the patient has been on the medication for a period of time. It is very important that the patients are educated about the potential side effects and possible decrease in the drug's efficacy. They should be able to recognize red flag signs of symptoms of each of these. They should understand the importance of follow-up visits and testing to evaluate their particular medication regime.

Discontinuation phase

The discontinuation phase of drug therapy is when a particular medication is stopped. Most psychiatric medications are not stopped abruptly, but require the dose to be slowly decreased over time. During the time the drug is being weaned off, the patient should be closely monitored for reappearance of the unwanted symptoms. By weaning off the medication, withdrawal symptoms can also be avoided. Some diagnoses, such as schizophrenia, require mediation to continue throughout the patient's life. Support, reassurance, and education are vital to the successful discontinuation of many psychiatric medications.

Tolerance, dependency, and withdrawal symptoms of medications

A person can develop a tolerance to a particular medication when that medication is used over a period of time. The effects of the medication diminish and can lead to a need to increase the dosage to achieve the same response. Sometimes dependency and withdrawal symptoms can be seen along with the development of tolerance. Dependency can be psychological or physical in nature. The withdrawal of this medication can produce stress or anxiety along with real physical symptoms. The medication will often have to be weaned by slowly decreasing the dosage. In severe cases, abrupt discontinuation of the medication can lead to death.

Ethnic, cultural, and gender considerations with drug therapy

Cultural and ethnic beliefs can affect an individual's attitudes and practices concerning health care. Communication and assessment of the patient can be complicated by language and social considerations. It may be difficult to get the patient to open up and verbalize their symptoms. The provider should be knowledgeable, respectful, and sensitive to an individual's cultural beliefs and how they affect their treatment regime. Along with the social considerations of different ethnic and cultural backgrounds come the biological differences. The biological differences between race, culture, and gender can affect the efficacy of the medication. There can be biologic, genetic, and hormonal differences that affect how a person responds to medications at a cellular level.

Drug therapy for children and the elderly

Medications can affect the very old, the very young, pregnant and breast-feeding women, and different cultures in a variety of ways. Dosages are usually less for the elderly population. Medical disease processes may affect the metabolism and clearance of many medications and they may also take many other medications that can lead to drug-drug interactions. Drug therapy in children will often require adult dosages due to their increased ability to quickly metabolize the medications. Children may also exhibit more unusual responses or side effects to drugs than adults and should be very closely evaluated and frequently assessed.

Pediatric pharmacology
There are a number of pediatric pharmacology concerns. Pediatric doses are calculated according to the child's weight in kilograms, but other factors may affect dosage. Weight is estimated by age (although actual weight is safer):

$$\text{50th percentile weight (kg)} = (\text{age} \times 2) + 9.$$

Only pediatric medications should be prescribed if possible. Adult pills, for example, should not be cut for use for a child as even small variations in dosage may have adverse effects. Dosages should always be checked. Drug therapy in children may sometimes require adult dosages due to the increased ability of children to metabolize the medications quickly. Children may also exhibit unusual responses (e.g., paradoxical effects) or side effects to drugs compared to adults and should be very closely evaluated and frequently assessed.

Gerontological pharmacology
A number of issues can affect gerontological pharmacology, which are listed below:
Antidepressants are associated with excess sedation, so typical doses are only 16%–33% of a younger adult's dose. Although selective serotonin reuptake inhibitors are safest, fluoxetine (Prozac) may cause anorexia, anxiety, and insomnia and should be avoided.
Older antipsychotics, such as haloperidol, have a high incidence of side effects. Atypical antipsychotics appear to be safer; risperidone (< 2 mg daily), for example, has the fewest adverse effects. The lowest possible dose should be tried first with careful monitoring of any antipsychotic.
Adverse effects of drugs are two to three times more common in older patients than younger patients, which is often related to polypharmacy.
Drugs may impact nutrition by impairing appetite. Interactions may also alter the pharmacokinetics of nutrients or drugs, interfering with absorption, distribution, metabolism, and elimination.

Administering medications

When administering medications, the nurse should verify the five rights (i.e., patient, medicine, dose, route, time). Medications in unit-dose packaging should be placed in medicine cups and the packaging opened in the patient's presence. Liquid medications should be carefully measured in appropriate medicine cups. Oral medications should be taken in the presence of nursing staff followed by at least 60 cc of fluid to ensure that the medications have been swallowed. Procedures may vary within different facilities. If hoarding is a problem, patients may be asked to open their mouths for examination after taking medications. If medications are mixed with food or fluids, this should first be discussed with the interdisciplinary team and documented as to reasons (e.g., confusion); this is done to avoid the legal implications of coercion as this practice may be misconstrued as administration of hidden medications.

Antipsychotic medications

Typical and atypical antipsychotic medications

With recent research and development of new antipsychotic medications, there has developed a need to differentiate between the older and newer drugs. The drugs originally utilized to treat psychosis are often referred to as the typical antipsychotic medications. These medications are also known as neuroleptics or major tranquilizers. Drugs of this class include medications such as Thorazine and Haldol. The newer medications created within the last 20 years are referred to as atypical antipsychotic medications. The newer drugs have fewer side effect and unwanted associated neurologic symptoms such as tardive dyskinesia. Drugs of this class include medications such as Risperdal and Zyprexa. The atypical class of medications is now considered the first-line drug therapy choice.

Symptoms affected by medications: The typical antipsychotic medications will only affect the positive targeted symptoms, while the newer atypical antipsychotic medications will affect both the positive and negative targeted symptoms. The positive targeted symptoms are associated with an excess of normal function and mainly affect the psychotic thinking processes and disorganization of speech, motor movements and social behaviors. Examples of these can include delusions, hallucinations, incoherence, catatonic motor movements, or unacceptable social behaviors. The negative targeted symptoms are associated with a reduction of normal function and mainly affect mood, cognition, and socialization. Examples of these can include a flat affect, a reduction in thought and speech, inability to focus or experience pleasure, or apathy.

Cardiovascular side effects

There are many different side effects that may occur with use of antipsychotic medications. One of the most dangerous side effects includes those involving the cardiovascular system. Symptoms can include orthostatic hypotension and ECG changes. Orthostatic hypotension is produced because certain antipsychotic medications bind with alpha adrenergic receptors. Medications such as chlorpromazine, thioridazine, and clozapine have been associated with causing orthostatic hypotension. The ECG changes that can occur include a prolonged Q-T interval within the QRS complex. Medications such as thioridazine and ziprasidone have been associated with this ECG abnormality.

Indication and mechanism of action

The most common indicator for the use of antipsychotic drugs is the treatment of psychosis. This class of medication is also used in the treatment of schizophrenia, organic brain syndrome, delusional disorders, agitation associated with the progression of Alzheimer's disease, substance-induced psychosis, severe depression with associated psychosis, and disruptive behaviors associated with dementia or delirium. The typical antipsychotic medications are postsynaptic dopamine antagonists with the new atypical class blocking serotonin as well and dopamine receptors. The difference in their mechanism of action results in a different patient response and targeted symptom treatment.

Unwanted weight gain

Certain antipsychotic medications can cause an increase in hunger and therefore lead to unwanted weight gain. The lower potency antipsychotics are more commonly associated with this side effect with clozapine and olanzapine as common culprits. Patients should be educated that increased weight leads to increased risks for cardiovascular disease and diabetes. They should be encouraged to start a diet and exercise program as soon as this side effect becomes evident. Alternative medications such as ziprasidone and quetiapine should be considered because they have shown no indication of causing unwanted weight gain.

Anticholinergic side effects
Anticholinergic side effects are due to the blocking of acetylcholine. These side effects can be seen with both typical and atypical antipsychotic medications. Symptoms can include dry mouth and mucous membranes, decreased gastric motility and constipation, urinary retention and/or hesitancy, blurry vision, confusion, or memory loss. These types of side effects can be seen with many psychiatric medications. The patient's should be reassured that many of these side effects are only temporary. They should be encouraged to perform good oral hygiene, use lip balm, eat a high fiber diet, and to postpone any eye exams for approximately 3 weeks after a consistent medication dosage has been determined.

Potential development of blood disorder
Blood disorders associated with the use of antipsychotic medications do not occur often but can be very dangerous. The use of clozapine has been associated with increased risk of developing what is called agranulocytosis. This is an acute reduction in the normal level of WBC's and neutrophils. Their reduction increases the risk for life threatening infections. They may need to be hospitalized so they can be closely monitored and placed in reverse isolation. Common symptoms include fever of unknown origin, malaise, sore throat, and mouth sores. The patient will need to have blood drawn to check these levels once a week for approximately the first 6 months and then every 2 weeks for the duration of the medication therapy. Prescriptions should only be given for one week at a time. Once clozapine has been stopped, blood samples should be checked for an additional 4 weeks. The patient should be educated to report any fever, sore throat, or mouth sores immediately and discontinue the medication until a CBC can be drawn.

Risk for seizures and water toxicity
In patients with undiagnosed underlying seizure disorder, the use of antipsychotic medications can lower their seizure threshold. This can lead to the onset of seizure disorder. Patients with already diagnosed seizure disorder should be very closely monitored for increased seizure activity. One of the more serious side effects associated with use of antipsychotic medications is water toxicity. This can develop over time and leads to ingestion of large quantities of water. The patient will develop polydipsia and polyuria and may appear puffy in the face or around the eyes. Hyponatremia will develop, which can cause confusion; agitation; abdominal distention; or if untreated, death. These patients should be weighed daily and serum sodium levels monitored closely.

Photosensitivity and pigment changes
Photosensitivity can occur while taking certain antipsychotic medications. Patient's using low-potency antipsychotics should be aware that they are at increased risk of developing severe sunburns or rashes related to sun exposure. They should be educated to wear sun block lotion or cover all exposed skin and to wear dark sun glasses when outdoors. Pigment changes can also occur with sun exposure. These areas of skin can become discolored due to pigment deposits and may range in color from orange to bluish grey. The face and neck areas are at the greatest risk for this discoloring. Patient's taking high doses of the drug thioridazine may experience pigment changes in the eyes called retinitis pigmentosa. This condition can lead to a severe decrease in vision. Recommended doses of thioridazine are 800mg/d or less.

EPS

Extrapyramidal symptoms (EPS) occur commonly with use of antipsychotic medications. There are three main syndromes that fall into this category. They include dystonia, parkinsonism, and akathisia. These symptoms usually develop early in treatment and resolve by approximately 3 months. Many times these symptoms are frightening to patients, causing them to stop their medications. They can also be confused with anxiety related symptoms. Assessment and symptom recognition are vital to the successful treatment of the patient. Some treatment options may include a reduction in the dosage of medication, a change to a different medication, or adding a new drug to specifically treat the symptoms. Patient reassurance, support, and education about these syndromes can help to decrease stress and anxiety.

NMS

Neuroleptic malignant syndrome (NMS) is one of the most serious complicating side effects associated with use of antipsychotic medications. This potentially fatal and rare condition can result with one single dosage of medication. The highest risk medications fall into the high-potency category. Symptoms occur acutely and can include high fever, tachycardia, diaphoresis, rigid muscles, shaking, incontinence, confusion and decreased level of consciousness, renal failure, and elevated CPK levels. It is very important to always monitor a patient's temperature with use of antipsychotics. The patient may require supportive care in the form of resuscitation, mechanical ventilation, hydration, and fever reducing actions. All antipsychotic drugs must be discontinued and the patient may be treated with dantrolene or bromocriptine. Development of this side effect does not exclude the patient from future treatment with antipsychotic medications.

Pseudoparkinsonism

With pseudoparkinsonism, many of the symptoms are the same as Parkinson's disease, but the cause is different. Parkinson's disease occurs due to the loss of dopaminergic cells, while pseudoparkinsonism is a medication induced state. Symptoms may include rigidity, slowing movements associated with akinesia, and tremors. Many times muscle rigidity is first noticed in the upper extremities. Increased salivation, mask-like facial expressions, and a decrease in reflexes or initiation of movements may also occur. Pseudoparkinsonism occurs more commonly in men and the elderly population. Symptoms usually appear within the first month of treatment and unfortunately there is usually no development of tolerance or resolution of symptoms. Treatment of symptoms with amantadine may help; however, the patient must have good renal function to take this medication.

> ➤ **Review Video:** Parkinson's Disease
> *Visit **mometrix.com/academy** and enter **Code: 110876***

Dystonia

Dystonia is a syndrome associated with EPS that can occur with the use of antipsychotic medications. This is often the first of the associated syndromes to occur and usually appears within the first few dosages of medication. Symptoms include spasms of the large muscle groups of the head, neck, and back. Patient complaints may also include a thick tongue or stiff neck. These symptoms can have an abrupt and painful onset. If untreated, this syndrome can lead to more severe symptoms, such as a protruding tongue, oculogyric crisis, torticollis, laryngopharyngeal constriction, or extreme abnormal posturing of the upper body. If the muscle spasms become sustained, this can lead to impaired respiratory status and a medical emergency. These symptoms are more often seen in children and young men.

Akathisia

The side effect of akathisia associated with the use of antipsychotic medications leads to an inability of the patient to remain still. They will often exhibit repetitive motions, such as pacing or rocking back and forth. They will often feel restless and the only way to relieve this restlessness is by moving. It is also possible for the individual to feel inner restlessness and not exhibit outward symptoms. They may be unable to relax and experience high levels of anxiety. Many times the patient will be unable to explain their need to move about. Akathisia symptoms can be difficult to treat. Limited success has been seen with use of beta-adrenergic blockers, anticholinergics, antihistamines, and low-dose antianxiety medications. The patient should be switched to an atypical antipsychotic. If unable to change medications the lowest effective dose of a typical antipsychotic can be used.

A complete baseline assessment is vital information to help differentiate between akathisia and an increase in psychotic symptoms. Akathisia can often be confused with agitation or an exacerbation of the patient's psychotic symptoms. Often the patient will have their medication dosages increased, only to find that there has been an increase in symptoms. Agitation associated with psychotic behavior does not usually just acutely appear after the initiation of antipsychotic medication. If possible, the provider should try to distinguish between muscle restlessness associated with akathisia or mental restlessness associated with agitation. The patient needs reassurance and validation that the symptoms are a treatable side effect of their medication.

TD

Tardive dyskinesia (TD) is a chronic syndrome that can develop as a result of the long term use of antipsychotic medications. The elderly population is at the highest risk for development of this syndrome. There is currently no effective treatment and the best defense is early detection and prevention of symptoms. Use of the lowest effective dosage of an atypical antipsychotic is often recommended for prevention. Frequent assessments for development of these symptoms are vital due to the fact that many of the patients are unaware that the symptoms may be occurring in the early phases. Symptoms can include involuntary movements of the face, such as tongue protrusion, lip smacking, blinking, grimacing, or chewing. Patients can also experience choreiform movements of the extremities and trunk of the body such as repetitive finger movements or irregular breathing patterns and swallowing air, which causes frequent belching and grunting to occur.

Medications for bipolar disorder

Mood stabilizing medications

Mood stabilizing medications are most commonly utilized to treat bipolar disorder. This disorder is characterized by recurrent periods of mania and if left untreated is associated with increased rates of morbidity and mortality. The goal of treatment with mood stabilizing medications is to prevent recurrence of acute episodes while functioning at an optimal level of production in daily life. Lithium remains the treatment of choice; however, some anticonvulsants such as carbamazepine and valproate have shown some mood stabilizing properties. In addition calcium-channel blockers have also been used in conjunction with other medication choices to control symptoms. FDA approved medications for treatment of bipolar disorder include lithium, olanzapine, and valproic acid.

Lithium

Required work-up: Lithium has a very narrow therapeutic window and toxicity is a medical emergency and can lead to death. It is cleared from the body by the kidneys and can negatively affect thyroid function. An initial assessment should include an evaluation of kidney function. This would be determined through a urinalysis (UA), BUN and creatinine levels, an electrolyte panel, 24-hour urine for creatinine clearance, screening for diabetes, hypertension, and any history of diuretic medications or over use of analgesics. Thyroid function must also be evaluated. A TSH, T3, T4, and free thyroxine index should be drawn. A complete physical along with a complete family and patient history should be obtained. Other tests should include a 12 lead ECK, fasting blood sugar, and CBC.

Indications and mechanism of action: Lithium is considered the gold standard in drug treatment for patients with mania. It helps control acute exacerbations of mania and provides long term stabilization of symptoms. It is also utilized for some depression symptoms, aggressiveness, or schizoaffective disorder. The exact mechanism of action is unknown; however, it is thought that lithium works to normalize the exchange of multiple neurotransmitters, such as dopamine, norepinephrine, serotonin, and acetylcholine. Lithium is transported across the cell membrane and is retained more readily than sodium within the cell. Therefore, physical symptoms that may decrease sodium levels, such as vomiting or excessive sweating, will affect lithium levels.

Toxicity: Lithium replaces sodium in the sodium-potassium pump within the body and is retained more readily than sodium within the cell. Therefore, any physical change that would affect sodium levels would affect lithium levels. Decrease in dietary sodium intake, vomiting, diarrhea, diaphoresis, fever, or greatly decreased fluid intake can lead to an increase in plasma lithium levels. The use of certain medications, such as loop or thiazide diuretics, ACE inhibitors, alcohol, carbamazepine, haloperidol, or NSAIDs, can also cause an increase in lithium levels. Lithium levels can also be decreased by increased dietary intake of sodium, caffeine, osmotic diuretics, or use of acetazolamide.

Because lithium has a very narrow therapeutic window, plasma levels must be frequently monitored. The normal therapeutic range is 0.6 and 1.4 mEq/L for adults. Lithium toxicity is an emergency and can lead to patient death. Plasma levels will usually decrease to an acceptable level within 48 hours after discontinuation of the medication; however, in severe cases involving acute renal failure, dialysis may be necessary. A complete initial assessment, ongoing assessments, frequent evaluations of lithium levels, and patient education are all an essential part of the treatment plan and prevention of toxicity. A patient must be able to tell the difference between side effects and symptoms of toxicity.

The symptoms associated with lithium toxicity can be similar to many of the side effects. It is vital that the patient and provider be well educated on the differences between the two. Early detection of toxicity can prevent devastating patient outcomes. Symptoms of mild toxicity associated with blood levels between 1.5 – 2.5 mEq/L can include severe vomiting and diarrhea, increased muscle tremors and twitching, lethargy, body aches, ataxia, ringing in the ears, blurry vision, vertigo, or hyperactive deep tendon reflexes. More severe symptoms associated with blood levels greater than 2.5 mEq/L can include elevated temperature, low urine output, hypotension, ECG abnormalities, and decreased level of consciousness, seizures, coma, or death.

Side effects and adverse reactions: There can be many side effects and adverse reactions associated with the use of lithium. As serum levels of lithium increase, so do associated side effects. If plasma levels are kept at the lower therapeutic end, many of the associated symptoms are mild and may resolve after a few weeks of treatment. Some of the side effects include the following: weight gain, fine motor tremors, fatigue, headaches, inability to concentrate, outbreaks of acne, or a maculopapular rash, GI upset, diarrhea, decrease in appetite, polyuria, polydipsia, or swelling. GI symptoms can be decreased if the dosage is taken with food or milk. Lithium is contraindicated in pregnancy, especially during the first trimester.

Nursing interventions side effects: Nursing interventions and patient education about these interventions can help ease some of the side effects associated with the use of lithium. For edema, elevate the hands or feet, monitor for weight gain, monitor I&O for decreased urine output, and monitor salt intake. For tremors, provide reassurance. Stress can increase the tremors. If the tremors interfere with daily functioning, notify the ordering provider. Mild diarrhea or GI upset can be decreased with smaller more frequent dosing of lithium taken with food. If diarrhea worsens, notify the healthcare provider and monitor for signs of toxicity. The patients experiencing the side effects of weakness, fatigue, and inability to concentrate will need reassurance that these symptoms usually resolve in a few weeks. Sugarless hard candy can help reduce symptoms of dry mouth or a metallic aftertaste. Encourage regular oral care to protect mucous membranes.

Anticonvulsants

Anticonvulsant medications are most commonly used to treat seizure disorder. However, they have also shown effectiveness in a reduction of mania symptoms associated with bipolar affective disorder. There are several anticonvulsant medications that are utilized in the treatment for mania. They include the following: valproic acid, gabapentin, carbamazepine, topiramate, lamotrigine and oxcarbazepine. These medications are often second-line drugs for patients unresponsive to lithium. Patients with mixed or dysphoric mania have been found to benefit most from use of anticonvulsants to treat their symptoms of high anxiety and agitation.

Carbamazepine

Carbamazepine (Tegretol) is considered to be a third-line medication choice for bipolar disorder. Divalproex and lithium are usually used in treatment before this medication choice. This medication can be added for use in combination medication therapy for bipolar disorder. Side effects can include sleepiness, vertigo, ataxia, blurred or double vision, GI upset, fatigue, or rarely causing a rash. This medication is metabolized by the CYP-450 enzyme found in the liver and can lead to dangerous interactions and decreased effectiveness of other anticonvulsants, anticoagulants such as Coumadin, or oral birth control pills. The use of this medication can lead to the very dangerous side effect of agranulocytosis, which is a decrease in the white blood cell count and can lead to fatal infections.

Divalproex

Divalproex (Depakote), a derivative of valproic acid, has the fewest side effects adverse reactions and the lowest potential for toxicity of all anticonvulsants used to treat bipolar disorder. This medication has become the first-line medication choice for treatment of bipolar disorder because of its low potential for toxicity and effective treatment in several subgroups of bipolar disorder. It is usually well tolerated by the patient with side effects including GI upset, tremors, drowsiness, headache, vertigo, and ataxia. It has also been associated with increased appetite and weight gain. The appearance of unexplained bruising, petechiae, or bleeding can indicate thrombocytopenia and the drug must be stopped. The most dangerous adverse side effect to this medication is severe liver damage. Liver function tests are obtained before starting the drug, then every 1-4 weeks for 6 months, followed by routine evaluations every 3-6 months throughout treatment. This medication is contraindicated during pregnancy.

Antidepressants

Indications for treatment

The main indicator for use of an antidepressant is simply depression. This can be further expanded to include major depression, atypical depression, and anxiety disorders. Depression type symptoms commonly include loss of interest in usual or pleasurable activities, decreased levels of energy, having a depressed mood, decreased ability to concentrate, loss of appetite, or suicidal thoughts. Antidepressants are also commonly used to treat anxiety disorders that include panic attacks, obsessive-compulsive disorder (OCD), social phobias, anxiety attacks, or posttraumatic stress disorder. They may also be beneficial in treating chronic pain syndromes, premenstrual syndrome, insomnia, attention deficit hyperactivity disorder, or bed wetting.

SSRIs

Selective serotonin reuptake inhibitors (SSRIs) prevent the reuptake of serotonin at the presynaptic membrane. This increases the amount of serotonin in the synapse for neurotransmission. This class of antidepressants has been shown to reduce depression and anxiety symptoms. Common side effects are usually short in duration and include headache, GI upset, and sexual dysfunction. They do not cause significant anticholinergic, cardiovascular, or significant patient sedation side effects. Examples of SSRIs include citalopram (Celexa), escitalopram (Lexapro), fluoxetine (Prozac), Fluvoxamine (Luvox), paroxetine (Paxil), and sertraline (Zoloft). These drugs are not highly lethal in overdose.

Tricyclic antidepressants

Side effects: Tricyclic antidepressants not only block the reuptake of serotonin and norepinephrine, they also act to block muscarinic cholinergic receptors, histamine H1 receptors, and alpha1 noradrenergic receptors. These receptors do not affect depression symptoms, but their blockade is implicated in some of the side effects associated with tricyclics. The blockade of the muscarinic receptors produces anticholinergic side effects such as dry mouth, blurred vision, constipation, urinary retention, and tachycardia. The blockade of the histamine receptors is associated with drowsiness, low blood pressure, and weight gain. The alpha1 noradrenergic receptor blocking action produces the side effects associated with orthostatic hypotension, vertigo, and some memory disturbances.

Mechanism of action and necessary evaluations: Most of the tricyclic antidepressants have very similar mechanisms of action and side effects. Although their exact mechanism of action is unknown, they are believed to act to inhibit the reuptake of both serotonin and norepinephrine. These drugs have a high first-pass rate of metabolism and are excreted by the kidneys. A complete physical and history should be obtained before starting a patient on tricyclic drugs. Because this class of antidepressants can cause death with an overdose, an initial suicide risk assessment must be obtained with continued assessments for this risk a necessity. This class of drug can cause a prolongation in the electrical conduction of the heart. Therefore, a baseline ECG should be performed in children, young teenagers, anyone with cardiac electrical conduction problems, and adults over age 40.

MAOIs

Side effects: Side effects associated with the use of monoamine oxidase inhibitors (MAOIs) are similar to many other antipsychotic medications. They can include symptoms such as GI upset, vertigo, headaches, sleep disturbances, sexual dysfunction, dry mouth, visual disturbances, constipation, peripheral edema, urinary hesitancy, weakness, increased weight, or orthostatic hypotension. The elderly population is at greatest risk for problems with orthostatic hypotension and should have lying, sitting, and standing blood pressure checks to monitor for this side effect. Orthostatic hypotension can lead to injuries related to falls such as fractures. The most dangerous side effect can be an extreme elevation in blood pressure.

Monoamine oxidase inhibitors (MAOIs) are associated with many different side effects; however, the most dangerous side effect is the development of a severe increase in blood pressure or hypertensive crisis. Hypertension can develop due to the presence of increased levels of tyramine. These levels increase because monoamine oxidase, which normally metabolizes tyramine, is inhibited. Increased levels of tyramine produce a vasoconstrictive response by the body that leads to increased blood pressure. Symptoms associated with hypertensive crisis can include severe occipital headache, palpitations, chest pain, diaphoresis, nausea and vomiting, flushed face, or dilated pupils. Complications associated with hypertensive crisis include hemorrhagic stroke, severe headache, or death. In depth patient education is vital and should include symptoms of hypertension, close monitoring of blood pressure, and low-tyramine diet.

Mechanism of action: The mechanism of action for monoamine oxidase inhibitors (MAOIs) is exactly what their name indicates. These drugs act to inhibit the enzyme monoamine oxidase (MAO). There are actually two of these enzymes, MAO A and MAO B, and this class of medication inhibits both. These enzymes act to metabolize serotonin and norepinephrine. By inhibiting the production of these enzymes, there are increased levels of serotonin and norepinephrine available for neurotransmission. Medications that selectively inhibit MAO B have no antidepressant effects and can be used to treat disease processes such as Parkinson's.

Diet restrictions: Monoamine oxidase inhibitors can lead to increased levels of tyramine in the nerve cell. These increased levels can lead to a dangerous and possibly fatal increase in blood pressure. Certain foods that contain tyramine should be avoided to help prevent hypertensive episodes. These foods include any cheeses except for fresh cottage, ricotta, processed cheese slices, or cream cheese, and any meat, fish, or poultry that has been improperly stored, fermented, or dried, including pepperoni, salami, summer sausage, pickled, or smoked fish. Other foods include fava or broad bean pods, sauerkraut, overripe fruit, banana peels, all tap beers, beef and chicken liver, any fermented product, products containing monosodium glutamate, or soybean condiments such as soy sauce. Red wine can produce the side effect of headache unrelated to hypertension and should also be avoided.

Calculating antidepressant doses

Antidepressants: Tricyclics and Heterocyclics	
Classes include the following: Tricyclics (amitriptyline, amoxapine, clomipramine, desipramine, doxepin, imipramine, nortriptyline, protriptyline, trimipramine) Heterocyclics (bupropion, maprotiline, mirtazapine, trazodone)	Doses are calculated according to a daily dosage range, which varies for different drugs (amitriptyline, 50–300 mg daily; nortriptyline, 30–150 mg daily, bupropion, 200–450 mg daily). The initial dose is usually given at a fairly low dose, depending on the degree of depression (somewhat higher for inpatients than outpatients) and may be given in a single dose or divided doses. Slow titration is necessary because response may take 1–4 weeks.

Antidepressants: Selective Serotonin Reuptake Inhibitors (SSRIs)	
Includes: Citalopram (Celexa) Escitalopram (Lexapro) Fluoxetine (Prozac) Fluvoxamine (Luvox) Paroxetine (Paxil) Sertraline (Zoloft)	Doses are calculated according to a daily dosage range, which varies for different drugs (citalopram, 20–40 mg; sertraline, 50–200 mg). The initial dose is usually low and titrated as necessary. For patients with comorbid anxiety, a low initial dose is essential. Because response often takes up to 4–6 weeks, the initial dose should not be increased for several weeks. If adverse effects occur, a lower dose should be given. If symptoms subside, the dose may be increased at a later time if necessary. If no response occurs after 4–6 weeks, then a different medication should be considered.

Monitoring antidepressants

Tricyclics and heterocyclics
Observe for toxicity.
Inform patients not to take with monoamine oxidase inhibitors.
Observe for decreased therapeutic response to hypertensives (e.g., clonidine, guanethidine).
Monitor other medications; patient should avoid other central nervous system depressants, including alcohol. Some medications potentiate the effects of tricyclics, including bupropion, cimetidine, haloperidol, selective serotonin reuptake inhibitors, and valproic acid.
Inform patient to avoid prolonged exposure to sunlight or sunlamps.
Administer major dosage of drug at bedtime if patient experiences drowsiness.
Monitor for sedation, cardiac arrhythmias, insomnia, gastrointestinal upset, and weight gain.

Selective serotonin reuptake inhibitors

Antidepressants: Selective Serotonin Reuptake Inhibitors (SSRIs)
Monitor for increased depression and suicidal ideation, especially in adolescents. Inform patients of the following: Smoking decreases effectiveness. Fatal reactions may occur with monoamine oxidase inhibitors. Taking SSRIs with benzodiazepines or alcohol has an additive effect. Some drugs, such as citalopram, may increase the effects of β-blockers and warfarin. Avoid cimetidine, which is prescribed for ulcers and gastroesophageal reflux disease, and St. John's wort. Inform patients of possible decreased libido and sexual functioning. Monitor for insomnia and gastrointestinal upset.

Antianxiety medication

Benzodiazepines
Indications for use: Benzodiazepines are the most commonly prescribed medications for anxiety. Some of the more commonly prescribed include chlordiazepoxide, lorazepam, diazepam, flurazepam, and triazolam. Benzodiazepines act to enhance the neurotransmitter GABA. This neurotransmitter inhibits the firing rate of neurons and therefore leads to a decline in anxiety symptoms. Indications for their use can include anxiety, insomnia disorders, alcohol withdrawal, seizure control, skeletal muscle spasticity, or agitation. They can also be utilized to reduce the

anxiety symptoms pre-operatively or before any other type of medical procedure such as cardiac catheterization or colonoscopy. This class of drug is also the treatment of choice for alcohol withdrawal.

Side effects: There are several common side effects associated with the use of benzodiazepines. One of the most common is the effect of drowsiness. Patients should be advised to use caution when operating motor vehicles or machinery. Activity will help decrease this effect. Other side effects include feelings of detachment, irritability, emotional lability, GI upset, dependency, or development of tolerance.

The elderly population is at high risk for development of dizziness or cognitive impairment, which places them at high risk for falls with associated injuries. When discontinuing a benzodiazepine after long term use, the drug should be weaned off to prevent withdrawal side effects.

Treatment of insomnia: Benzodiazepines are used to treat insomnia because of their sedative-hypnotic effects. There are three different types of insomnia, which include the inability to fall asleep, inability to stay asleep, or the combination of both. Many times insomnia can be helped by a change in habits or talking about worries or stress the patient may be experiencing. When using a sedative-hypnotic to treat sleep disturbances, the medication should have rapid onset and allow the patient to wake up feeling refreshed instead of tired and groggy. When administered at HS, most benzodiazepines will produce a sleep inducing effect and should be used on a short-term basis.

Evaluation of a patient before starting antianxiety and sedative-hypnotic medications
Antianxiety medications are indicated when symptoms of anxiety are out of proportion for the situation. Physical disease processes or illness should be ruled out first before determining that the anxiety should be treated as a psychiatric problem. Disease process such as hypothyroid, hypoglycemia, cardiovascular disease, or pulmonary disease can produce anxiety symptoms. Other medications or substance abuse should also be ruled out as possible causes. Many times anxiety occurs along with other psychiatric disturbances; therefore, the patient should be screened for other disorders such as depression or schizophrenia. Many times the anxiety symptoms will resolve if the main psychiatric disorder is treated appropriately.

Buspirone
Due to the addictive potential of benzodiazepines, the use of nonbenzodiazepines to treat anxiety has increased. One of the most commonly used nonbenzodiazepine medications is the drug buspirone. This medication is highly effective in treating anxiety and its associated symptoms such as insomnia, poor concentration, tension, restlessness, irritability, and fatigue. Buspirone has no addiction potential, is not useful in alcohol withdrawal and seizures, and is not known to interact with other CNS depressants. Because it may take several weeks of continual use for the effects of this drug to be realized by the patient, it cannot be used on an as needed basis. Buspirone does not increase depression symptoms and therefore is useful in treating anxiety associated with depression. Side effects associated with medication can include GI upset, dizziness, sleepiness, excitement, or headache.

Calculating doses and monitoring antianxiety agents
Antianxiety Agents Classes include the following:
- Antihistamines (hydroxyzine)
- Benzodiazepines (alprazolam, bromazepam, chlordiazepoxide, clonazepam, clorazepate, diazepam, lorazepam, oxazepam)
- Tranquilizers (meprobamate)

- Azapirones (buspirone)

Doses are calculated, according to a daily dosage range, which varies for different drugs (e.g., alprazolam, 0.75–4 mg daily; diazepam 4–40 mg daily). The usual procedure is to start with a low initial dose and then slowly increase the strength every 3–4 days or longer if the response is inadequate. Buspirone has a delayed onset, so the initial response does not occur for up to 2 weeks.

- Administer with food or milk, but avoid grapefruit juice.
- Inform patient that abrupt discontinuation may cause life-threatening effects.
- Observe for reduced anxiety, exacerbation of depression, or paradoxical excitement.
- Monitor for orthostatic hypotension and blood dyscrasias (e.g., sore throat, bruising, bleeding).
- Provide ice chips, sugarless gum, and hard candy for dry mouth.
- Provide stool softeners for constipation.
- Inform patient to avoid central nervous system depressants, such as alcohol.

Stimulants

Stimulant medications are utilized to treat attention deficit hyperactivity disorder, narcolepsy, and obesity that persist despite trying other treatment options. They are also used along with other medications to treat fatigue common in depression or other mood disorders. These stimulants lead to an increased level of catecholamines in the synapse. They increase the levels released as well as block their reuptake. They mainly affect dopamine and norepinephrine levels. Side effects of these medications can include decreased appetite, sleep disturbances, vertigo, irritability, GI upset, headache, palpitations, tachycardia, irregular heart rate, dry mouth, or constipation.

Trial period for new medication

When initiating any sort of pharmaceutical treatment for mental disorders, it is important to have an adequate trial period for new medication before switching to alternative therapies due to unresponsiveness. Generally speaking, a medication, such as an antipsychotic is tested for 8 weeks before switching. However, 4–6 weeks is sufficient for stimulants before opting for a second-line treatment. Before switching medications, one should check with a pharmacist to ensure the dose of the current therapy has been optimized. It is not uncommon for agents to be prescribed in doses that fail to optimize the drug. Drug optimization may occur at either a lower or higher dose for an individual patient than the dose commonly prescribed. Dose optimization is one of the many reasons why upward and downward titrations are important.

CAM

Complementary and alternative medicine (CAM) focuses on the whole person including not just the physical aspects but the spiritual and psychosocial aspects as well. This approach utilizes many different philosophies and therapies that work together to help incorporate all aspects of the person as a whole in the healing process. Alternative medicine is used alone, whereas complementary medicine is used in conjunction with conventional Western medicine. There are five major categories of complementary and alternative medicine. These include alternative medical systems, mind-body interventions, biologically based therapies, manipulative and body-based methods, and energy therapies.

Mind-body interventions

The domain of mind-body interventions utilized with complementary and alternative medicine (CAM) incorporates a variety of techniques designed to improve the mind's ability to alter physical symptoms of diseases. This system believes that the mind can help keep the body healthy. Some of these interventions, such as support groups and cognitive-behavioral therapy, are now utilized in more mainstream Western style medicine. Other examples of these types of interventions are still considered to belong to the realm of CAM and can include meditation; guided imagery; relaxation techniques; aromatherapy; hypnosis; prayer; and art, humor, light, music, or dance therapy. Many of these therapies are widely utilized as alternative treatments or in complement with conventional medicine to treat chronic pain.

Alternative medical systems

Alternative medical systems are complete systems of theory and practice. These systems have come into being and progressed apart from the more conventional biomedical approach. Many of these systems were already in existence for hundreds or thousands of years before the inventions of conventional medicine. Examples of these systems include traditional oriental medicine, Ayurveda, homeopathy, and naturopathy. Ayurveda promotes good health and disease prevention through a healthy lifestyle. This system utilizes massage, meditation, yoga, healthy diet, and herbal medicine. Homeopathy operates under the belief that the body can heal itself. This system believes that if a certain substance causes symptoms, then giving the same substance in small diluted doses the body can cure the symptoms by enhancing the body's natural healing processes. Naturopathic medicine also believes the body can heal itself and promotes health and healing through the use of organic food, exercise and leading a well balanced healthy lifestyle.

Manipulative and body-based methods and energy therapies

The domain of manipulative and body-based methods in complementary and alternative medicine is based upon the manipulation and movement of parts of the body. Some examples of this domain include massage therapy, chiropractic or osteopathic manipulation, and reflexology. The domain of energy therapies focuses on energy fields. Within this domain there are two different types of energy fields. The first type is biofield therapy which affects the energy fields that surround the body or are derived from within the body. Examples of biofield therapy include qi gong, Reiki, and therapeutic touch. The second type of energy field is electromagnetic based therapies, which use energy from sources outside the body. Examples of these types of therapies include pulsed fields, magnetic fields, alternating current, or direct current fields.

Biologically based therapies

The domain of biologically based therapies in complementary and alternative medicine (CAM) utilizes products found in nature. These practices include the use of interventions and products that may be sometimes utilized by conventional medicine, such as the use of dietary supplements. Other examples of these products can include herbal treatments or special nature based diets. Some of these therapies, such as use of shark cartilage to treat cancer, are controversial and lack any scientific evidence to support their use.

Acupuncture

One of the main uses for acupuncture is for the treatment of pain. This treatment originated in China in the sixteenth century and has been recognized by the World Health Organization to assist with symptom relief of over 30 disease processes or conditions. This treatment involves the insertion of stainless steel needles into 14 acupoints found along the body's energy channels or meridians. The belief is that this treatment restores the balance of energy within the body. The insertion of the needles induce an ache within the stimulated muscle, which then sends a message to the central nervous system to release endorphins, which block pain, along with serotonin and norepinephrine.

St. John's wort for depression

The use of complementary and alternative medicine for the treatment of depression is very common. One of the most widely utilized and studied herbal therapies for the treatment of depression is St. John's wort or hypericum. This particular herb is widely utilized to treat depression symptoms in both the United States and in European countries. It has shown some effectiveness in treating moderate depression, anxiety disorder, insomnia, or seasonal affective disorder. Medical providers should be aware if the patient is taking this herb due to its contraindications with many commonly prescribed medications such as birth control pills, statins used to treat hyperlipidemia, protease inhibitors, antineoplastics, SSRIs, anticonvulsants, theophylline, and anticoagulants such as Coumadin.

Pain

Psychological impact

Pain is now recognized as a complex human experience that not only involves the physiological aspect but also involves a powerful psychological emotional response. The patient's response to pain is influenced by cognitive abilities; culture; and socioeconomic, environmental, motivational, and behavioral factors. The pain as described by the patient is subjective in nature; however, many of the physical signs, such as change in vital signs, can be measured objectively. Everyone experiences pain differently. The impact of pain has led to many different treatment approaches including the use of medications or alternative therapies.

Beginning steps in evaluating and treating pain

The first step in the treatment of pain is to establish a diagnosis for the source of the pain. The next step is to determine a goal for pain control. The patient may need to realize that complete pain resolution is not possible and pain reduction is a more realistic goal. Next, other associated symptoms, such as depression or anxiety, should be treated.

Some of the first line pharmacological treatments for pain include analgesics, NSAIDs such as acetaminophen or ibuprofen, local anesthetics, topically applied agents, neuroleptics, corticosteroids, baclofen, calcitonin, or benzodiazepines such as clonazepam. Medications for pain maintained per the sympathetic nervous system could include propanolol or nifedipine.

Second level of treatment

If all of the initial treatment options have failed for the patient experiencing pain, then a second level treatment approach should be initiated. This begins with the utilization of antidepressant medications along with counseling support. The use of a transcutaneous electrical nerve stimulation (TENS) device can be utilized to attempt to control pain. Tricyclic antidepressants, MAOIs, SSRIs, and anticonvulsants such as carbamazepine or neurontin can also be effective in helping the individual achieve their best level of pain control. Second line opioid analgesics such as codeine, Demerol, or morphine can be utilized if initial pain medications were not effective. Many individuals also consider herbal and alternative medical therapies.

<u>Third level of treatment options</u>
For the patients that do not achieve a tolerable level of pain through the first two treatment steps the third level should be evaluated. This level can be utilized in conjunction with any portion of the first two levels that achieved some relief. This allows the provider to build upon any positive outcomes to help reach the goal. Adrenergic agents, TENS units, and additional psychological counseling and support can be added to the treatment regime. Medications such as clonidine, naloxone infusions, mexiletine, and diphenhydramine can have additive properties to enhance the actions of other medications or be utilized to treat unwanted side effects.

<u>Fourth level of treatment options</u>
If the patient has still not achieved an acceptable level of pain control through the first three steps, there are still options available to try to reach their pain goal. Many of these patients will need psychotherapy to help them address the psychological impact and symptoms they may be experiencing. They may need to reevaluate their pain goal to include a realistic expectation for their personal situation. They may need reassurance to help reduce anxiety levels and reinforcement of new learned coping and adaptation behaviors. Other options can include possible ablation for specific sources of pain, neuroblockade procedures such as epidural steroid injections or nerve root blocks, or spinal cord stimulation through neurostimulator implants. If the patient has not found some success with any treatment options, then a complete psychological evaluation for severe depression and risk for suicide should be performed.

Psychoeducation for bipolar disorder and schizophrenia

Psychoeducation, often part of cognitive-behavioral therapy, involves teaching individuals about their disease to help them manage symptoms and behavior.
- Bipolar disorder: Individuals are taught to understand the patterns of their disease and the triggers of mood changes so they can seek appropriate medical help. Additionally, they are taught to use self-monitoring tools, such as a daily record, to determine patterns of activity, such as sleeping, so they can maintain as consistent a schedule of eating, sleeping, and engaging in physical activities as possible; consistency tends to reduce unstable mood swings.
- Schizophrenia: Individuals must be taught about their disease and the effects of medications. Because medication may not eliminate all symptoms, such as hearing voices, individuals are taught methods to test reality to determine if their perceptions are correct.

Evidence based practice

Evidence based practice is developed by the using the best evidence provided from systematic research performed for the purpose of evaluating patient care practices. This information provides a method to examine patient interventions and determine their effectiveness. The nurse can no longer rely on opinion-based information or theoretical frameworks alone to determine nursing interventions. Nursing is now responsible for seeking out research literature, utilizing critical thinking skills to evaluate the research findings, and then applying the findings to actual practice guidelines.

Crisis intervention

Crisis intervention occurs when the goal of treatment is to return the individual to their pre-crisis state. This treatment course usually lasts six weeks or less and is geared towards assisting the individual to create new coping mechanisms and adaptive behaviors. Social and cultural influences can greatly affect the ability and ways in which individuals deal with and work through a crisis. There may be preconceived ideas and beliefs about asking for and accepting assistance from others. It is very important to consider the age of the individual when assessing the need for particular crisis interventions. The needs of an elderly adult will be different than those needs of a child.

Conflict resolution

When attempting to resolve conflict between two or more individuals, the desired outcome is a feeling by each party of getting what they wanted out of the situation. Resolving conflict should include the following steps:
- Assisting the involved parties with problem identification.
- Ascertaining the expectations for each person involved.
- Identification of each person's specific interests within the conflict.
- Assisting the parties with creating ideas to help resolve the conflict.
- Assisting the parties in bringing together a situation where everyone can feel happy about the outcome.

With the first step in the conflict resolution process, the problem is identified. The parties are each allowed their opportunity to discuss what they think is wrong. This portion of the resolution process may become emotional and involve angry outbursts. With the second step, ascertaining expectations occurs when each party identifies exactly what they want. With the disclosure of these expectations, a sense of trust can begin to evolve. The nurse will need to remain objective and respectful to everyone involved during this phase. With the next phase, the nurse will need to determine if anyone has unspoken objectives or interests that could slow down the resolution progress. Everyone needs to be honest about what they want and need. In the final steps, everyone should work together to create and then compromise together to reach a resolution that works for everyone.

Behavior modification

Behavior modification is a type of systematic therapy that works towards the goal of replacing maladaptive behaviors with positive behaviors. This type of therapy can be utilized with individuals, groups, or entire communities. The hope of this approach is to get rid of the unwanted behaviors by utilizing positive reinforcement directed towards the desired behaviors. By utilizing positive reinforcement, the participant will want to repeat the good behaviors to gain the reward. These new behaviors will then become habit over time and will replace the old behavior. This type of therapy can be very effective with eating disorders, smoking cessation, or addictions.

ECT

Electroconvulsive therapy (ECT) is a treatment in which the use of a brief electrical shock is utilized to induce a seizure. Although it is not certain exactly how ECT works, it is believed that the seizure acts to alter certain electrochemical processes in the brain. ECT is not for everyone. Psychiatrists only administer this procedure to selective patient populations. ECT is recommended for individuals with severe depression that is unresponsive to medications or accompanied by suicidal ideations, psychosis, insomnia, homicidal ideations, or guilt and hopelessness. It is also recommended for schizophrenia or mania that is unresponsive to medications. It may also have some limited indications for use in catatonia, schizoaffective disorder, Parkinson's disease, or the individual in which certain medications are contraindicated. Use of ECT on the elderly population should be performed with great caution due to the coexistence of many contraindicated disease processes with this population. This population often has preexisting heart disease.

Before preparing for electroconvulsive therapy (ECT) the individual must first have a complete history and physical. This should include lab tests, EKG, and careful blood pressure evaluation for hypertension. The individual must be physically capable of tolerating the procedure. An anesthesiologist will also be consulted to evaluate for any contraindications to the use of anesthesia. After the procedure the individual will be taken to a recovery area where they will be monitored and the anesthetic is allowed to wear off. The patient usually begins to awaken 5-10 minutes after the procedure is completed. A short period of confusion lasting up to a few hours is not uncommon. Once completely awake, the patient may then dress, eat, and return home or to their room in the hospital.

Electroconvulsive therapy (ECT) is performed in a hospital setting. The individual may be inpatient or outpatient. ECT is performed up to 3 times per week with the total number of treatments ranging from 6 to 12. ECT is administered in the morning with the patient having been NPO to reduce the risk of vomiting and subsequent aspiration. The treatment is performed by a psychiatrist with an anesthesiologist present to administer short-acting anesthesia and muscle relaxant intravenously. The procedure itself takes approximately 10-15 minutes. Electrode pads are placed on the side of the head and the shock, lasting 1-2 seconds, can be administered unilaterally or bilaterally causing a brief seizure. The seizure usually lasts 30-60 seconds and is monitored by use of an EEG. A few minutes after the procedure is completed the patient begins to awaken.

Informed consent
An informed written consent must be obtained prior to the use of electroconvulsive therapy (ECT). This involves using clear and understandable language to educate the person about ECT, including what to expect before, during, and after the procedure; any benefits, risks, or side effects; how many treatments are expected; and any optional treatments available. Any and all questions are encouraged and clearly answered. A simple and concise video may also be a very useful educational tool to assist the individual in understanding what to expect with ECT. The individual should be updated on the progress of the treatments with each procedure and may withdraw consent to continue at any point during the course of treatment. If the person is unable to make decisions for him or herself, most local laws provide for the court to appoint a legal guardian to provide consent.

Potential risks
The risks associated with ECT are the same as many other medical procedures involving anesthesia. There are also risks involved with the introduction of an electrical shock into the body. The pre-procedural history and physical are very important in determining any preexisting contraindicated medical conditions such as heart disease, cardiac arrhythmias, pulmonary disease, central nervous system problems, hypertension, or previous reaction to anesthesia. The ECT may cause an increase in heart rate and blood pressure and could in rare cases, as in any medical procedure, lead to death.

<u>Side effects</u>

The side effects associated with electroconvulsive therapy (ECT) can originate from the administration of the electrical shock, the anesthesia, or more likely from a combination of both. Immediately after the treatment side effects may include headaches, transient confusion, muscle soreness, nausea, vomiting, or jaw pain. ECT can also cause some memory loss. This side effect may worsen over the course of treatment and may include retrograde amnesia, causing partial or complete memory loss of events occurring days, weeks, months, or occasionally years before the procedure. Memory loss during the actual time of the treatments may also occur. For most people, this amnesia will resolve within a few months after treatment has ended.

Single-session therapy

Single-session therapy is the most frequent form of counseling because individuals often attend only one session for various reasons even if more are advised. Individuals may not have insurance or believe that one session is sufficient. Sessions typically last 1 hour. The goal is to identify a problem and reach a solution in one session. The therapist serves as a facilitator to motivate the individual to view the problem as part of a pattern that can be changed and to identify a solution. The therapist may use a wide range of techniques that culminates in a plan for the individual (e.g., homework exercises) so the individual can begin to make changes.

Solution-focused therapy

Solution-focused therapy aims to find methods that are effective and those that are not and to identify areas of strengths so they can be used in problem solving. The premise of solution-focused therapy is that change is possible but that the individual must identify problems and deal with them in the real world. This therapy is based on questioning to help the individual establish goals and find solutions to problems:

- Pre-session: The patient is asked about any differences he or she noted after making the appointment and coming to the first session.
- Miracle: The patient is asked if any "miracles" occurred or if any problems were solved, including what, if anything, was different and how this difference affected relationships.
- Exception: The patient is asked if any small changes were noted and if there were any problems that no longer seemed problematic and how that manifested.
- Scaling: The patient is asked to evaluate the problem on a 1–10 scale and then to determine how to increase the rating.
- Coping: The patient is asked about how he or she is managing.

ERP for obsessive-compulsive disorder

Exposure and response/ritual prevention (ERP) is a type of therapy used to treat obsessive-compulsive disorder (OCD). ERP helps the patient learn to reduce anxiety by not performing ritualistic behavior. The goal is to habituate the person to the anxiety associated with an act so that it lessens and the ritual stops. Steps include the following:

- Psychoeducation: ERP begins with education about the nature of OCD and ritualistic behavior.
- Ritual/fear analysis: Fact-finding may be carried out in one or two sessions, during which a fear hierarchy is outlined regarding obsessional material starting with those that cause low anxiety and building to those that cause extremely high anxiety.

- Exposure and response/ritual prevention: Exposure begins with small steps. For example, if a person is obsessed with germs, a first step might be to touch a tissue that touched a toothpick that touched a dirty tissue. The response/ritual prevention part is to avoid washing hands after touching the tissue. This may be done repeatedly to desensitize the person before moving to a high-anxiety item on the fear hierarchy.

Group therapy

<u>Form and purpose</u>

Group Therapy Classified According to Form	
Homogeneous	Members chosen on a selected basis, such as abused women
Heterogeneous	An assortment of individuals with different diagnoses, ages, and genders
Mixed	A group that shares some key features, such as the same diagnosis, but differs in age or gender
Closed	A group in which new members are excluded
Open	A group in which the members and leaders change

Group Therapy Classified According to Purpose	
Task	Emphasis on achieving a particular assignment
Teaching	Developed to inform, such as teaching the rules of the unit
Supportive/ therapeutic	Assisting those who share the same experience to learn mechanisms to cope with trauma and to overcome the problem, such a group for battered women
Psychotherapy	Helping the patient reduce psychological stress by modifying behavior or ideas

Group development

<u>Pre-group phase</u>
The group process is very similar to the individual process in therapeutic communication. The group process has a beginning, middle, and end. The group can move through one phase and enter another, or regress back to the previous phase.
When a new member is added or conflict arises within the group, the phase can be altered. When beginning a group, certain criteria should be determined. These criteria should include a common goal, purpose or outcome, the meeting location or space, actual group members, and will the group be open or closed to addition of new members during the process. Group member selection is critical to the success of the group as a whole. The members should have a common purpose and potential for cohesiveness. The dynamics and interactions between group members will determine the success of the group.

<u>Beginning stage</u>
The beginning or initial phase of group development allows for the group to make introductions and begin to learn about each other and the leader. The group members may feel anxiety, fear, or distrust and may not reveal many of their true feelings. In the beginning of the phase the group members will often communicate very politely and be considerate of all members of the group. Often the group members will settle into particular roles. This phase then progresses into a period of conflict. Issues of who is powerful or who has dependency issues within the group may lead to struggles between group members. The leader will have to undertake the job of allowing the group members to discuss their hostilities and conflicts with each other as well as those with the leader

themselves. By the end of this phase, the group should be more cohesive and share a more positive bond. They should be ready to move into the working phase of the group process.

Working phase

During the working phase of the group process the members continue to form a more stable bond with each other. They share feelings and ideas and are moving towards their common outcome and purpose. Certain ritualistic norms may emerge and the group itself may form a particular personality. The leader may take on a different role and act more as a resource person for the group. However, they will continue to keep the group focused on their purpose and guide them forward. The group may at times still experience some degree of conflict or resistance from certain members as they move through this phase. By the end of this phase, the group should have a sense of pride about their accomplishments and they should have made great strides toward their goal achievement.

Termination stage

During the termination stage of the group process the members will physically separate and group meetings will come to an end. If the process was closed to new members, then the group will separate as a whole. If the process was open to new members, then the group members may separate individually. If the group has been successful, members may express feeling of sadness and loss and may start to make plans for meetings after the resolution of the group. These meetings often fail to occur and the leader should realize these plans are part of the process of letting go of the group. During this time, the group should undergo self evaluation and determine goal achievement. If successful, the group members should be able to apply their newly learned coping behaviors to their changing life situations.

PCIT

Parent–child interaction therapy (PCIT) is designed for preschool children with conduct disorder or oppositional defiant disorder. Sessions are usually 1 hour a week for 10–16 weeks. The therapist observes the parent–child interaction from outside the room (usually with a two-way mirror) and provides feedback. PCIT has two phases:

- Child-directed interaction: Parents learn specific skills to use when engaging children in free play, including reflecting a child's statements and describing and praising appropriate behavior while ignoring undesirable behavior. The goal is to strengthen the parent–child bond and eliminate undesirable behavior.
- Parent-directed interaction: During this phase, positive behaviors are increased and undesirable behaviors are decreased. Parents learn to give clear commands, provide consistent reinforcement, and use time out for noncompliance.

Incredible Years Program

The Incredible Years Program for conduct disorder and oppositional defiant disorder has both a child (ages 4–7) and a parent component:

- Child: "Dinosaur school" is a group of children (about six children) who attend 2-hour weekly sessions for about 17 weeks. Videos and life-sized puppets are used to demonstrate ways of dealing with interpersonal problems, such as making friends, empathizing, coping with teasing, and resolving conflicts. Children practice social skills and are rewarded for positive social skills. Parents receive weekly updates and are asked to reward children for positive social skills.

- Parent: Parents meet in groups (about ten parents) for 2-hour sessions for 22 weeks. Parents view seventeen videos modeling appropriate methods for dealing with problem behavior and discuss them in the group. Parents learn to initiate nonthreatening play sessions, use positive reinforcement and consistent limit-setting, and learn strategies for dealing with problem behavior, such as time-outs.

PSST and PMT

Problem-solving skills training (PSST) is designed for children 7–13 years old to address antisocial behavior, conduct disorder, and oppositional defiant disorder. Parents of these children can take a parent management training (PMT) course simultaneously.
- PSST: Children attend 50-minute individual weekly sessions for 25 weeks. The therapist presents problem situations similar to those faced by the child and then helps the child to evaluate the situation, develop goals, and alternate goals for dealing with these situations. As homework, children are assigned "super solver" tasks in which they use skills learned in therapy in real-life situations. Parents learn to assist the child in using new strategies.
- PMT: Parents attend a total of sixteen sessions of 2 hours each over a 6–8-month period. Parents learn techniques for managing their child's behavior, such as reinforcement, shaping, and time-outs. The therapist uses a variety of teaching methods, including instruction, modeling, and role-playing.

MST

Multisystemic therapy (MST) is a family-focused program designed for adolescents (11–17 years of age) with antisocial and delinquent behaviors. The primary goal is collaboration with the family to develop strategies for dealing with the child's behavioral problems. Services are delivered in the family's natural environment rather than at a clinic or office with frequent home visits, usually totaling 40–60 hours over the course of treatment. Sessions are daily initially and then decrease in frequency. A variety of different therapies may be used, including family therapy, parent training, and individual therapy. Therapists use different approaches but adhere to basic principles, including focusing on the strength of the systems, delivering appropriate treatment for developmental level, and improving family functioning. The goals of therapy are to improve family relations and parenting skills, to engage the child in activities with nondelinquent peers, and to improve the child's grades and participation in activities, such as sports.

FFT

Functional family therapy (FFT) is designed for adolescents (11–17 years of age) with antisocial behavior. FFT uses the principles of family systems theory and cognitive-behavioral therapy and provides intervention and prevention services. While the therapy has changed somewhat over the past 30 years, current FTT usually includes three phases:
- Engagement/motivation: The therapist works with the family to identify maladaptive beliefs to increase expectations for change, reduce negativity and blaming, and increase respect for differences. Goals are to reduce dropout rates and establish alliances.
- Behavior change: The therapist guides the parents in using behavioral interventions to improve family functioning, parenting, and conflict management. Goals are to prevent delinquent behavior and build better communication and interpersonal skills.

- Generalization: The family learns to use new skills to influence the systems in which they are involved, such as school, church, or the juvenile justice system. Community resources are mobilized to prevent relapses.

HRT

Habit reversal therapy (HRT), a form of cognitive-behavioral therapy, is used to help people with tic disorders and for those with impulse control disorders, such as trichotillomania. A number of steps are involved, which are listed in the following chart:

Awareness	The patient must pay attention, as behaviors are often unconscious. This often involves keeping a detailed log of the behavior, including time; duration; activity during the episode; and emotional state before, during, and after these behaviors.
Identification of triggers	The log and patient interviews help to identify triggers to help patients understand when they are at risk of the behavior and how to use stimulus control to prevent the behavior or to avoid triggers.
Assessment	The patient begins to identify feelings (negative or positive) associated with the behavior and the reason for it.
Competitive response	The patient carries out another action to compete with the urge to carry out the behavior, thereby preventing it.
Assessment of rationalizations	The patient must confront the rationalizations used to allow the behavior to continue.
Mindfulness	The patient learns that it is not necessary to give in to the urge to carry out the behavior as urges often are of short duration.

Therapy for obsessive-compulsive disorder

Therapy for obsessive-compulsive disorder aims to develop expression of thoughts and impulses in a manner that is appropriate:

Behavioral therapy (most successful)	Combined exposure with training to delay obsessive responses; best used in conjunction with pharmacotherapy Steady decrease of rituals by exposure to anxiety-producing situations until patient has learned to control the related obsessive compulsion Reduction of obsessive thoughts by the use of reminders or noxious stimuli to stop chain-of-thought patterns, such as snapping a rubber band on the wrist when obsessive thoughts occur
Family therapy	Primary issues include the following: Helping the family to avoid situations that trigger OCD response Pointing out the tendency of family members to reassure the patient, which is apt to support the obsession Introducing family strategies, which involve the following: Remaining neutral and not reinforcing through encouragement Avoiding trying to reason logically with the patient
Pharmacologic therapy	FDA-approved medications for OCD: clomipramine (Anafranil), sertraline (Zoloft), paroxetine (Paxil), fluoxetine (Prozac), and

	fluvoxamine (Luvox)

Therapy for post-traumatic stress disorder

Individuals with post-traumatic stress disorder (PTSD) are usually treated with antidepressants, mood stabilizers, or antipsychotic drugs, depending on their symptoms, but one of the following therapies is essential:

- Cognitive-behavioral therapy (CBT): Individuals learn to confront trauma through psychoeducation, breathing, imaginary reliving, and writing; they are taught to recognize thoughts related to their trauma and attempt a method of coping, such as distraction and self-soothing.
- Eye-movement desensitization and reprocessing: This form of CBT requires the individual to talk about the experience of trauma while keeping the eyes and attention focused on the therapist's rapidly moving finger. (There is no clear evidence this is more effective than standard CBT.)
- Family therapy: PTSD impacts the entire family, so counseling and classes in anger management, parenting, and conflict resolution may help reduce family conflict related to the PTSD.
- Sleep therapy: Individuals may fear sleeping because of severe nightmares. Sleep therapy teaches methods to cope with nightmares through imagery rehearsal therapy and relaxation techniques.

ACT

Acceptance commitment therapy (ACT) approaches behavioral change from a different perspective than conventional CBT. Patients are encouraged to examine their thought processes (cognitive defusion) when undergoing episodes of anxiety or depression. They identify a thought, such as "People think I am ugly," and then analyze whether or not this is true, listing evidence, and then evaluating whether or not the anxiety is decreased after this evaluation   process. Eventually, this process becomes automatic, eliminating the need to write everything down. Mindfulness is a basic concept of ACT, and patients are encouraged to examine their values and control those things that are under their control, such as their facial expression or actions. ACT represents (A) accepting reactions, (C) choosing a direction, and (T) taking action to effect change.

CBT

Cognitive-behavioral therapy (CBT) focuses on the impact that thoughts have on behavior and feelings and encourages the individual to use the power of rational thought to alter perceptions and behavior. This approach to counseling is usually short-term, about twelve to twenty sessions, with the first sessions used to obtain a history, the middle sessions used to focus on problems, and last sessions used to review and reinforce. Individuals are assigned "homework" during the sessions to practice new ways of thinking and to develop new coping strategies. The therapist helps the individual identify goals and then find ways to achieve those goals. CBT acknowledges that all problems cannot be resolved, but one can deal differently with problems. The therapist asks many questions to determine the individual's areas of concern and encourages the individual to question his or her own motivations and needs. CBT is goal-centered so each counseling session is structured toward a particular goal, such as coping techniques. CBT centers on the concept of unlearning previous behaviors and learning new ones, questioning behaviors, and doing homework. Different approaches to CBT include Aaron Beck's cognitive therapy, rational emotive behavior therapy, and dialectic behavior therapy.

Aaron Beck's cognitive therapy

Aaron Beck discovered that during psychotherapy patients often had a second set of thoughts while undergoing "free association." Beck called these "automatic" thoughts, which were labeled and interpreted, according to a personal set of rules. Beck called dysfunctional automatic thoughts "cognitive disorders." Beck identified a triad of negative thoughts regarding the self, environment, and world. The key concepts in Aaron Beck's cognitive therapy include the following:

- Therapist/patient relationship
- Therapy is a collaborative partnership. The goal of therapy is determined together. The therapist encourages the patient to disagree when appropriate.
- Process of therapy
- The therapist explains the following: The perception of reality is not reality. The interpretation of sensory input depends on cognitive processes. The patient is taught to recognize maladaptive ideation, identifying the following: Observable behavior, Underlying motivation, His or her thoughts and beliefs. The patient practices distancing the maladaptive thoughts, explores his or her conclusions, and tests them against reality.
- Conclusions
- The patient makes the rules less extreme and absolute, drops false rules, and substitutes adaptive rules.

Albert Ellis's rational emotive therapy

Key concepts of Albert Ellis's rational emotive therapy include the idea that people control their own destinies and interpret events, according to their own values and beliefs.

ABC therapy	Activating event, belief, and consequences (emotional or behavioral)
Irrational beliefs	Something should be different. Something is awful or terrible. One cannot tolerate something. Something or someone is damned or cursed.
"Musturbatory" ideologies	I must do well and win approval, or I am a rotten person. You must act kindly toward me, or you are a rotten person. My life must remain comfortable, or life hardly seems worth living.

Therapy consists of detecting and eradicating irrational beliefs, as follows:

- Disputing: detecting irrationalities, debating them, discriminating between logical and illogical thinking, and defining what helps create new beliefs
- Debating: questioning and disputing the irrational beliefs
- Discriminating: distinguishing between wants and needs, desires and demands, and rational and irrational ideas
- Defining: defining words and redefining beliefs

Dialectical behavioral therapy for borderline personality disorder

Dialectical behavioral therapy was developed for the treatment of patients with borderline personality disorder (BPD). In therapy, the nurse/therapist helps patients to change behavior by replacing dichotomous thinking that paints the world as black or white with rational (dialectical) thinking. This therapy is based on the premise that patients with BPD lack the ability to self-regulate, have a low tolerance for stress, and encounter social and environmental factors that impact their behavioral skills. Therapy includes the following:

Cognitive-behavioral therapy (once a week) focuses on adaptive behaviors that help the patient to deal with stress or trauma. Therapy focuses on a prioritized list of problems: suicidal behavior, behavior that interferes with therapy, quality of life issues, post-traumatic stress response, respect for self, acquisition of behavioral skills, and patient goals.

Group therapy (2.5 hours a week) helps the patient learn behavioral skills, such as self-distracting and soothing.

MET for substance abuse

Motivational enhancement therapy (MET) is a nonconfrontational, structured approach to treatment for substance abuse that is usually done in four sessions. MET helps motivate the patient to change, accept responsibility for change, and remain committed to change. The MET therapist guides the patient through different stages of change:

- Pre-contemplation: Patient does not wish to change behavior.
- Contemplation: Patient considers positive and negative aspects of drug or alcohol use.
- Determination: Patient makes a decision to change.
- Action: Patient begins to modify behavior over time (2–6 months).
- Maintenance: Patient remains abstinent.
- Relapse: Patient begins the cycle again. Relapses are common.

The therapist questions, compliments, and supports the patient but avoids criticizing, labeling, or directly advising the patient. Patients, especially those who have failed previous attempts to stop using, require much encouragement. A pretreatment assessment is completed, and the patient is provided with a written report at the first meeting. The therapist uses eight strategies during sessions, eliciting statements of self-motivation; listening empathetically; questioning; providing feedback; providing affirmation; handling or preventing resistance by reflecting, amplifying, or changing focus; reframing; and summarizing.

Visualization to treat anxiety disorders

Visualization (therapeutic imagery) is used to treat anxiety disorders primarily for relaxation, stress reduction, and performance improvement. Visualization may be used in conjunction with many other types of therapy, such as exposure therapy, which can be very stressful for some people. Visualization strives to create a visual image of a desired outcome in the mind of the patient when he or she imagines him- or herself in that place or situation. Intense concentration helps to block feelings of anxiety. For example, if the focus is on reducing anxiety, the mind focuses on that goal of therapy. All of the senses (e.g., looks, smells, feelings, sounds) may be used to imagine the feeling of relaxation in a certain place.

CBGT for social phobias

Cognitive-behavioral group therapy (CBGT) for social phobias is a form of exposure therapy done in a group environment, usually limited to about six patients with one or (preferably) two therapists to monitor and guide group exercises. Having an equal mix of men and women is preferred because social phobias often involve male–female interactions. Patients with different types of fears are appropriate for the group because they complement each other during therapy. The initial sessions involve psychoeducation about phobias and basic instruction in cognitive restructuring, including identifying automatic thoughts and discussing how they are errors in thinking. During exercises, such as speaking in front of the group, patients are asked to express their automatic thoughts and discuss them. The subjective units of distress rating scale (0–10 scale of distress) is used throughout exercises with patients giving their score every minute. Each patient is provided with individualized homework. Sessions are usually weekly for 2–3 hours for 12–24 weeks.

Patient-provider relationship

Working phase
The second phase of the patient-provider relationship is the working phase. During this time the patient will identify and evaluate specific problems through the development of insight and learn ways to effectively adapt their behaviors. The provider will assist the patient in working through feelings of fear and anxiety. They will also foster new levels of self-responsibility and coping mechanisms. The development of new and successful ways of approaching problems is the goal of this phase. The provider may often face resistance by the patient to move through this phase, and by utilizing different communication techniques may help to assist the patient in moving forward.

Introductory phase
The first thing the health care provider should do when meeting a patient is to find out why they are there. This initial phase provides a time for the provider and patient to get to know each other. There is no definite time frame and this phase can last for a few minutes to a few months. There are certain goals that should be accomplished during this time. The provider and patient should develop a mutual sense of trust, acceptance, and understanding. They may enter into a contract with each other. They will need to determine expectations, goals, boundaries, and ending criteria for the contract. This initial phase often involves obtaining the patient's history, their account of the problems, and developing a general understanding of the patient.

Termination phase
The final stage of the patient-provider relationship is the termination or resolution phase. This phase begins from the time the problems are actually solved to the actual ending of the relationship. This phase can be very difficult for both the patient and the provider. The patient must now focus on continuing without the guiding assistance of the therapy. The patient will need to utilize their new found approaches and behaviors. This time may be one of varying emotions for the patient and they may be reluctant to end the relationship. They may experience anxiety, anger, or sadness. The provider may need to guide the patient in utilizing their new found strategies in dealing with their feelings about the termination of the relationship. Focus should be placed on the future.

Verbal communication

Verbal communication is achieved through spoken or written words. This form of communication represents a very small fraction of communication as a whole. Much information achieved verbally may be factual in nature. Communication occurs along a two way path between the nurse and the provider. One limitation of verbal communication can be different meanings of words in different ethnic and cultural populations. The meanings may differ in denotative, actual meaning, and/or connotative, implied meaning, of the words. The use of words may differ depending upon personal experiences. The patient may assume the provider understands their particular meaning of the word.

<u>Silence and listening</u>
Silence and listening are very effective during verbal communication. Silence allows the patient time to talk and formulate ideas and responses. It is an intentional lull in the conversation to give the patient time to reflect. Listening is more active in nature and the provider lends attention to what the patient is communicating. There are two different types of listening. Passive listening allows the patient to speak without direction or guidance from the provider. This form of listening does not usually advance the patient's therapy. Active listening occurs when the provider focuses on what is said in order to respond and then encourage a response from the patient.

Non-verbal communication

Non-verbal communication occurs in the form of expressions, gestures, body positioning or movement, voice levels, and information gathered from the five senses. The non-verbal message is usually more accurate in conveying the patient's feeling than the verbal message. Many patients will say something quite different than what their non-verbal communication indicates. Non-verbal communication may also vary by cultural influences. The health care provider must be aware of these cultural differences and respect their place within the therapy. The provider should utilize positive, respectful, non-threatening body language. A relaxed, slightly forward posture with uncrossed arms and legs may encourage communication.

<u>Space zone boundaries and touch</u>
Space and touch as non-verbal forms of communication can vary greatly depending upon social or cultural norms. Space can provide information about a relationship between the patient and someone else. Most people living in the United States have four different areas of space. Intimate space is less than 18 inches, personal space is 18 inches to 4 feet, social-consultative space is 9 to 12 feet, and public space is 12 feet or more. Observations concerning space and the patient's physical placement in a setting can give a great deal of insight into different interpersonal relationships. Touch includes personal or intimate space with an action involved. This fundamental form of communication can send very personal information and communicate feelings such as concern or caring.

<u>Vocal cues, action cues, and object cues</u>
There are many different types of non-verbal behaviors. There are five main areas of non-verbal communication. They include vocal cues, action cues, object cues, space, and touch. Vocal cues can involve the qualities of speech, such as tone and rate. Laughing, groaning, or sounds of hesitation can also convey important communication. Action cues involve bodily movements. They can include things such as mannerisms, gestures, facial expressions, or any body movements. These types of movements can be good indicators of mood or emotion. Object cues include the use of objects. The patient may not even be aware that they are moving these objects. Other times the patient may choose a particular object to indicate a specific communication. This intentional use of an object can be less valuable than other forms of non-verbal communication.

Therapeutic communication

<u>Empathy</u>
Empathy is perhaps one of the most important concepts in establishing a therapeutic relationship with a patient, and it is associated with positive patient outcomes. It is the ability of one person to put themselves in the shoes of another. Empathy is more than just knowing what the other person means. The provider would seek to imagine the feelings associated with the other person's

experience without having had this experience themselves and then communicating this understanding to the patient. Empathy should not be confused with sympathy, which is feeling sorry for someone. The provider should also be aware of any social or cultural differences that could inhibit the conveyance of empathy.

Rapport and validation

Communication between the health care provider and the patient can be improved by establishing rapport and validating certain information. Establishing rapport with a patient involves achieving a certain level of harmony between the provider and the patient. This is often achieved through the establishment of trust through conveying respect, nonbiased views, and understanding. By establishing rapport, the provider helps the patient feel more comfortable about sharing information. Validation requires the provider to use the word "I" when talking with the patient. It evaluates one's own thoughts or observations against another person's and often requires feedback in the form of confirmation.

Open-ended statements and reflection techniques

Broad open-ended statements allow the patient the opportunity to expand on an idea or select a topic for discussion. This type of communication allows the patient to feel like the provider is actually listening and interested in what they have to say. It also helps the patient gain insight into emotions or situations. Reflection conveys interest and understanding to the patient. It can also allow for a time of validation so the provider can show that they are actually listening and understanding the shared information. It involves some minimal repetition of ideas or summing up a situation. These ideas or summaries are directed back to the patient often in the form of a question.

Restating and clarification techniques

Restating and clarification are verbal communication techniques that the provider may use as part of therapeutic communication. Restating involves the repetition of the main points of what the patient expressed. Many times the provider will not restate everything but narrow the focus to the main point. This technique can achieve both clarification of a point and confirmation that what the patient said was heard. Clarification involves the provider attempting to understand and verbalize a vague situation. Many times a patient's emotional explanations can be difficult to clearly understand and the provider must try to narrow down what the patient is trying to say.

Groups

A group is a gathering of interactive individuals who have commonalities. Interventions through group sessions can provide an effective treatment opportunity to allow for growth and self development of the patient. This setting allows the patients to interact with each other. This allows the patients to see the emotions of others such as joy, sorrow, or anger and to receive as well as participate in feedback from others in the group. The group can be very supportive and thrive in both inpatient and outpatient settings. The one thing the group cannot lack is definite leadership and guidance from the health care provider. The provider must guide those members of the group in facilitating therapeutic communications.

Detrimental techniques

Techniques that are detrimental to establishing a trusting therapeutic relationship include giving advice, challenging the patient's communications, or indicating disapproval. Giving advice includes telling the patient what they should do in a particular situation. This does not allow the patient to develop the ability to solve their own problems and may not always be the right answer. Challenging occurs when the patient's thoughts are disputed by the provider. This communication only serves to lower the patient's self-esteem and create an environment of distrust between the patient and the health care provider. Disapproval occurs when the provider negatively judges the patient's beliefs or actions. This again serves to lower patient self-esteem and does not foster their ability to solve their own problems or create new coping abilities.

Professional boundaries

Professional boundaries can be difficult to establish as part of the delivery of care, especially with diverse populations because the therapist may unknowingly violate personal or spiritual values. Diverse groups include, for example, homeless, abused, or immigrant populations. It is very important that therapists remain cognizant of the potential to abuse a position of power because patients and their families are dependent on the therapist or because language differences or cultural constraints may prohibit patients from being able to state their concerns. A relationship with an individual must be caring but at the same time professional and nonjudgmental. The needs of the patient or family must always be considered, and this may mean using a translator to ensure that the individual or family is taking an active role in the plan of care or making referrals to other health care professions.

Sexual behavior
When a nurse is in the position of "authority" in relation to a patient, the responsibility to maintain professional boundaries rests with the nurse; however, the boundary separating the nurse and the patient is sometimes not easily defined. A potential boundary issue may include sexual behavior. It is inappropriate for nurses to engage in sexual relations with patients, and if the sexual behavior is coerced or if the patient is cognitively impaired, it is illegal. However, more common violations, especially with older or impaired adults, include exposing a patient unnecessarily, using sexually demeaning gestures or language (e.g., off-color jokes), harassment, or inappropriate touching. Touching should be used with care, such as touching a hand or shoulder. Hugging can easily be misconstrued.

Gifts
Over time, patients may develop a bond with nurses they trust and may feel grateful to the nurse for the care provided and want to express thanks, but the nurse must make sure to maintain professional boundaries. A potential boundary issue is when patients offer gifts to nurses to show their appreciation; however, older adults, especially those who are weak, ill, or cognitively impaired, are easily manipulated. For example, patients may offer valuables or be manipulated into giving large sums of money. Small tokens of appreciation that can be shared with other staff, such as a box of chocolates, are usually acceptable (depending on the policy of the institution), but almost any other gifts (e.g., jewelry, money, clothes) should be declined: "I am sorry; that is so kind of you, but nurses are not allowed to accept gifts from patients." Declining a gift may relieve the patient of feelings of obligation.

Coercion
Power issues are inherent in matters associated with professional boundaries. Physical abuse is both unprofessional and illegal, but behavior can easily border on abuse without the patient being physically injured. A potential boundary issue is the use of coercion. Nurses can easily intimidate patients into having procedures or treatments they do not want. Patients have the right to refuse treatment. Difficulties arise with patients who are cognitively impaired, in which case, another responsible adult is designated to make decisions; however, every effort should be made to gain patient cooperation. Forcing the patient to do something against his or her wishes borders on abuse and can sometimes degenerate into actual abuse if the coercion is physical.

Attention

Nursing is a giving profession, but nurses must temper giving with recognition of professional boundaries. A potential boundary issue is giving patients too much attention, so that they become overly dependent and obligated. Patients have many needs, especially the elderly or those with personality disorders; as acts of kindness, nurses often give them extra attention but may become overly invested in the patients' lives. While this may benefit a patient in the short term, it can foster a relationship of increased dependency and obligation that does not resolve the long-term needs of the patient. Making referrals to the appropriate agencies and collaborating with the family to find ways to provide services are more effective. Becoming overly invested may be evident by nurses showing favoritism or spending too much time with certain patients while neglecting other duties. On the other end of the spectrum are nurses who are disinterested and fail to provide adequate attention to the patient's detriment. Lack of adequate attention can lead to outright neglect.

Personal information

When preexisting personal or business (dual) relationships exist, other nurses should be assigned to care for patients whenever possible; this may be difficult in small communities, however. Nurses must strive to maintain a professional role separate from the personal role and respect professional boundaries. Nurses must respect and maintain the confidentiality of their patients and family members, but they must also be very careful about disclosing personal information; sharing personal information establishes a social relationship that interferes with the professional boundaries that are necessary between patient and nurse. When the nurse divulges personal information, he or she may become vulnerable to the patient, an unhealthy role reversal.

Psychiatric and mental health programs

A variety of psychiatric and mental health programs are available and should be evaluated, according to the needs of the individual patient. Inpatient programs provide a secure environment and comprehensive care, often with psychologists, psychiatrists, occupational therapists, social workers, and other allied health personnel. Programs may be tailored to one specific type of patient (e.g., criminally insane, substance abusers) or to a general population. They may offer short-term or long-term care. Outpatient programs provide assessment and treatment, such as group therapy, cognitive-behavioral therapy, and family therapy. Programs may be community-based, targeting specific groups of people, such as alcoholics or the homeless. Partial/day hospitalization programs provide daily inpatient care during prescribed hours (e.g., 8 a.m. to 3 p.m.) as well as outpatient services. The stay is usually short-term (1–2 weeks) and may serve as a transition from inpatient to outpatient care.

Therapeutic milieu

The therapeutic milieu setting is a stable environment provided by an organization to assist in a treatment plan. The main purposes of a milieu are to teach individuals certain social skills and to provide a structured environment that promotes interactions and personal growth along with attempting to control many types of deviant or destructive behaviors. There are five main components that the milieu should include in their therapy. These components include containment, support, validation, structure, and involvement. Through the use of these components, the therapeutic milieu can help the individuals achieve their highest level of functioning.

Containment component

The containment component in a milieu involves the actual physical safety of the participants. It provides a safe clean physical environment as well as providing food and some medical care. The actual environment will often be very comfortable with colorful walls, pictures, and comfortable chairs and couches. They are allowed a certain freedom of movement throughout this environment. Many times the participants will work to help maintain a clean and functioning environment. They may perform certain tasks or chores to help with the upkeep of the milieu. This containment will provide a feeling of safety and trust for the individual.

Structured component

The structured component in the milieu lies hand in hand with consistency. The milieu provides a place with consistent staff members, physical surrounds, and limits on behavior. This predictability allows the participants to feel safe and secure and to know what to expect. This environment also provides structure through providing an environment where the participants can interact with a purpose. These purposes can range from daily tasks and chores to the different roles they may assume within various meetings. Through acceptance of this consistent and structured environment, the individual can begin to achieve some level of self-responsibility and consequences for their actions.

Support component

The support component in a milieu comes directly from the staff members involved in the milieu. Their goal is to help the participants have increased self-esteem through creating an environment of acceptance for all individuals. They provide a safe and comfortable atmosphere, therefore decreasing anxiety levels. Encouragement, empathy, nurturing, reassurance, and providing physical well-being for each participant will help increase their feelings of self worth. Consistency in attitudes and actions by all staff members are very important in the success of this setting. By providing this type of environment, the milieu will assist them in their abilities to gain new healthy relationships and appropriate interactions with others.

Involvement component

The involvement component of the milieu is the development of a sense of open involvement for each patient from the staff members. The staff should convey their desire to be personally involved with each patient through both their actions and attitudes. They should encourage the patients to communicate with them openly about feelings and experiences. This sense of individual interest and involvement will help to increase the patient's sense of self-worth and self-esteem. The staff members should encourage patient involvement through encouraging patient-lead group sessions and activities. By becoming involved, the patients have opportunity to practice new social skills such as working together with others, learning to compromise, and dealing with conflict. The hope of involvement is to achieve the goal of appropriate social interactions for each patient.

Validation component

The validation component of the milieu is the recognition of each patient as an individual. The staff members should convey respect and consideration for each and every patient. This respect and consideration should be shown through acts of kindness, empathy, nonjudgmental attitude, and acceptance of each individual for who they are. In a milieu, each patient contributes through responsibilities and involvement in many decision making processes. Through these actions, the patients should begin to feel some self-responsibility and with this new sense of responsibility comes validation for their individuality and humanity.

Monitoring and observation

Monitoring, directly watching patients in psychiatric and mental health care, varies, depending on the type of facility and the patient's condition. It is primarily used to ensure safety. Monitoring can include the following:

- Routine checks are done at prescribed times (e.g., every 15 minutes), or continuous observation may be necessary.
- Security personnel (e.g., in emergency departments) may monitor patients to ensure patient and staff safety.
- Audio/video monitoring is sometimes used, but patients and families must be aware that this kind of monitoring is in place; it must not violate privacy, and monitors and audio speakers must not be accessible to nonauthorized individuals. Regulations regarding audio/video recordings may vary from state to state.

Observation is an ongoing process that involves observing the patient's behavior and nonverbal actions (e.g., posture, eye contact, expression, clothing, tone of voice) during communication. Observation helps to determine which issues are important to the patient, the types of questions to ask, the patient's perceptions, and the interpretation of messages.

Five rights of delegation

Before delegating tasks, the nurse should assess the needs of the patients and determine the tasks that need to be completed, assuring that he or she can remain accountable, can supervise the task appropriately, and can evaluate effective completion. The five rights of delegation include the following:

- Right task: The nurse should determine an appropriate task to delegate for a specific patient.
- Right circumstance: The nurse must consider the setting, resources, time and safety factors, and all other relevant information before determining the appropriateness of delegation.
- Right person: The nurse is in the right position to choose the correct person (by virtue of education and skills) to perform a task for a given patient.
- Right direction: The nurse provides a clear description of the task, the purpose, any limits, and expected outcomes.
- Right supervision: The nurse is able to supervise, intervene as needed, and evaluate performance of the task.

Patient safety issues

Professional assault response
A protocol for a professional assault response should be established at all mental health facilities because statistics show that 75% of mental health staff experience a physical assault; most injuries are incurred by nursing staff caring for violent patients. Assaults may occur in both psychiatric units and emergency departments, where security staff may also be assaulted. Additionally, patients may be victims. Common injuries include fractures, lacerations, contusions, and unconsciousness from head injuries. Victims are at risk for psychological distress and post-traumatic stress syndrome, so a prompt response is critical. The assault response should include the following:

- Routine assessment of patients for violent or aggressive tendencies
- Protocol for managing violent or aggressive patients

- Physical assessment and medical treatment as needed for injuries
- Completion of an incident report by those who were involved or who observed the incident
- Psychological intervention, including individual counseling sessions and critical incident stress management, which requires a response team that includes staff members who are trained to deal with crisis intervention (e.g., psychologists, psychiatrists, nurses, peer counselors, social workers)

CISM

Critical incident stress management (CISM) is a procedure to help people cope with stressful events, such as disasters, to reduce the incidence of post-traumatic stress disorder.
Defusing sessions usually occur very early, sometimes during or immediately after a stressful event; these sessions are used to educate actively involved personnel about what to expect over the next few days and to provide guidance about how to handle stress reactions. Debriefing sessions usually follow in 1–3 days and may be repeated periodically as needed. These sessions may include personnel who were either directly involved or indirectly involved. People are encouraged to express their feelings and emotions about the event. The six phases of debriefing include introduction, fact sharing, discussion of feelings, describing symptoms, teaching, and reentry. Critiquing the event or attempting to place blame is not part of the CISM process. Follow-up is done at the end of the process, often after only a week, but this time period, of course, varies.

Contraband and unsafe items

State regulations identify contraband and unsafe items that are prohibited from mental health and correctional facilities; however, each facility must develop site-specific restrictions and protocols for responding to contraband and unsafe items. Contraband may include the following:
- Alcohol or products (mouthwash) that contain alcohol
- Drugs, including prescription, over-the-counter, and illicit drugs
- Poisonous and toxic substances
- Pornographic or sexually explicit material
- Food (hoarded or excessive)
- Depending on the type of facility or patients, a wide range of items may be considered unsafe. These often include the following:
- Knives, scissors, sharp instruments, and razor blades
- Flammable materials, such as lighter fluid and matches
- Breakable items, such as glass and mirrors
- Dangerous materials (which might be used for a suicide attempt), such as belts (over 2 in wide), large buckles, rope, electrical cords (i.e., over 6 feet in length), and wire
- Potential weapons, such as pens (except felt point), pencils, and plastic bags
- Electrical equipment, such as fans and recording devices

Collaboration in developing and updating a care plan

One of the most important forms of collaboration in developing and updating a care plan is between the nurse and the patient and his or her family, but this type of collaboration is often overlooked. Nurses and others on the health care team must always remember that the point of collaborating is to improve patient care; this means that the patient and the patient's family are central to all planning. Including the family is time-consuming initially, but asking and evaluating what the patient and family want can provide valuable information that can facilitate planning and improve the allocation of resources. Families, and even young children, often feel validated and more positive toward the medical system when they are included in the decision-making process.

Impact of poverty on access to care

Poverty often limits access to care. Many patients with psychiatric and mental health problems are ineligible for Medicaid, lack other health insurance, or do not have the financial resources to pay for care. Free clinics and mental health programs are sometimes available, especially in urban areas, but many people do not have access to or money for public transportation to go to medical visits, especially in rural areas, and cannot afford medications. Additionally, rates of depression are higher among those with low income, and depression often prevents people from seeking help. Employers may not allow people to take time off from work when practices are open to provide care, or patients cannot afford to lose income; thus, most medical care is provided by emergency departments when a crisis arises.

Cultural beliefs about the causes of mental illness

The following are some cultural beliefs about the causes of mental illness:
- African American: Spiritually out of balance
- Arab Americans: Punishment from Allah, sudden onset of fear, or pretense
- Cambodians: Brutalities related to the Khmer Rouge
- Chinese: :Evil spirits or lack of emotional harmony
- Cubans: Hereditary condition or result of severe stress
- Filipinos: Disharmony between individuals and the spirit world
- Haitians: Supernatural events
- Japanese-Americans: Evil spirits cause lack of self-control, punishment for behavior, or failure to lead a good life
- Mexican-Americans: Combination of factors, including God, interpersonal relationships, humoral aspects (blood/body fluids), and spirituality
- Native Americans: Violations of taboos, ghosts, and lack of harmony between the individual and the natural world
- Puerto Ricans: Heredity and post suffering
- Russians: Stress or a new environment
- Southeast Asians: Evil spirits or spells
- Vietnamese: Haunting by spirits (ancestral) and disruption of individual harmony

Gay, lesbian, bisexual, and transgender patients

Gay, lesbian, bisexual, and transgender patients often experience hostility and discrimination because of their sexual identification. Some experience anxiety and stress when coming to terms with their sexuality or when "coming out" to family or friends. Increasingly, adolescents are self-identifying as homosexual, some as early as age 12, and they may face intense pressure from family and peers. Homosexual or transgender military personnel must deal with the fear of being identified and losing their careers. Hate crimes against homosexual or transgender individuals continue. Children of gay or lesbian parents may face discrimination as well. While some religious groups and therapists recommend "reparation" therapy to convert homosexuals to heterosexuals, the American Psychiatric Association opposes such therapy, and evidence suggests that it is virtually never successful and can be damaging psychologically. The nurse must respect the individual's sexual identification, remain supportive, and should be knowledgeable about issues that are important to gay, lesbian, bisexual, and transgender patients. The rights and needs of partners should also be respected.

Restrictive measures

The use of restrictive measures is a last resort in most patient settings. When utilized, these measures are to promote patient safety. The most common types of restrictive measures include physical restraints and seclusion. Every patient is entitled to being treated with the greatest personal respect and dignity. When a patient's activity is restricted very careful monitoring is required. Specific documentation on the patient's well being should be performed per the facilities policy and usually includes a description of what occurred and physical monitoring of the patient while in restraints. If restrictive measures have to be utilized, staff members should have attempted and documented any and all other attempts to de-escalate the situation. These restraint techniques should only be utilized during the time that the patient is considered dangerous.

Seclusion

Seclusion involves separating the patient from others by placing them in an environment where they are unable to leave. The patient is usually placed in this environment against their will in order to protect the patient or others from harm. This particular type of restraint is viewed negatively, is associated with negative patient outcomes, and is rarely utilized. A seclusion room would have padded walls and no furniture. There would be nothing in this environment that the patient could utilize to injure themselves or someone else. Once a patient has been placed in seclusion, they must be observed continuously.

Restraints

Restraints are considered to be the most restrictive of all measures and should only be utilized if all other alternative measures have failed. There are two main types of restraints: chemical and physical. Chemical restraints involve the use of medications to manage a patient's behavior problem. This type of restraint often inhibits their physical movements and is used only when absolutely necessary to prevent injury. This medication is not utilized on a regular basis. Physical restraints involve the use of a person physically restraining a patient or the use of a mechanical device to restrict movement. These restraints not only restrict the physical movements in an area, but can also restrict their access to other parts of their own body or nearby equipment. Physical restraints are very difficult for patients to remove on their own.

Impact of being homeless on access to care

The homeless population has disproportionate rates of serious mental illness, estimated at about 40%–45%, such as schizophrenia and bipolar disorder, complicated by substance abuse. The need for adequate housing is an ongoing problem with homeless patients. Once released from inpatient care services, the homeless often return directly to the streets or to shelters. They are often victimized by others, suffer relapses, or engage in substance abuse in an attempt to self-medicate. The homeless often resist treatment (sometimes not believing they are ill), fail to keep appointments, or lack transportation or money for transportation. They may have no money for medication, may not qualify for assistance, or may be reluctant to deal with government agencies to gain assistance.

Alternative housing arrangements and residential services

The need for adequate housing is an ongoing problem with psychiatric patients. Many of these patients are homeless and once released from inpatient care services do not have anywhere to live. A safe and affordable option is vital to the success of their treatment. Many of these patients have a relapse of their mental illness or suffer medical illnesses, incarceration, or abuse by others. The most common housing available includes group homes, such as personal care homes or board and care homes; therapeutic foster care; and supervised apartments. Many of these provide some type of rehabilitation and/or support services.

Therapeutic foster care homes and supervised apartments

Therapeutic foster care provides for the patient in a home setting with a family that is trained to care for high needs patients. This training includes medication education, crisis management, and disease education. The foster family supervises all aspects of the patients care and incorporates them into the structure of the home. Many times the patients will share household work and may attend daytime care programs. This level of care is available for both children and adults. Supervised apartments provide each patient with their own apartment. Patients may either live alone or share the apartment with a roommate. They are responsible for the upkeep of the apartment and are independent in their self-care needs. The apartment is supervised by staff members that regularly check on the residents to ensure that they are doing well and following prescribed medication regimes.

Personal care homes and board-and-care homes

Personal care homes are located in homes in residential communities. These homes can usually provide supervised care for up to approximately 10 individuals. Services often include supervision of medication regimes, provision for transportation needs, meals, and assistance with activities of daily living. Many of these patients are elderly or suffer mild intellectual disability or psychiatric illness. Board-and-care homes are similar to personal care homes; however, there is little assistance with activities of daily living. Many of these patients can provide their own self care with little supervision. These homes are usually larger in size and accommodate up to 150 individuals. Both of these residential services are licensed by the state.

Professional Role

Accreditation

Mental health care facilities are highly regulated and evaluated by several different accrediting bodies. The process of accreditation occurs when a facility is determined to be providing acceptable quality care based upon certain established standards. Nursing is critically evaluated during the accreditation process and is vital in meeting the agency accreditation standards. When a facility is accredited, this information is made public so that the consumer will be aware of which institutions meet the acceptable standards of care. It is also necessary for a facility to maintain to receive third party reimbursement for services.

There are many different organizations that provide accreditation to mental health care delivery systems. One of the most important accrediting bodies is the Joint Commission on Accreditation of Healthcare Organizations (JCAHO). This is the accrediting body for hospitals throughout the United States. The accrediting body of the Centers for Medicare and Medicaid Services (CMS) determine accreditation standards for facilities seeking Medicare or Medicaid reimbursement. Community mental health facilities do not seek accreditation from JCAHO or CMS. These outpatient facilities seek accreditation from the Commission on Accreditation of Rehabilitation Facilities.

Standards of care

The practice of mental health nursing is guided by the standards of care. Professional nursing groups such as the American Nurses Association (ANA), American Psychiatric Nurses Association and the International Society of Psychiatric-Mental Health Nurses set the standards of care and identify the nursing process as the basis for nursing interventions and clinical decisions. The standards of care are based upon the nursing process, which includes the patient assessment, diagnosis, outcome identification, planning, implementation, and evaluation. Each nurse is responsible for being aware of their practice standards and being able to function at this level.

NDNQI

The National Database of Nursing Quality Indicators (NDNQI) is a database containing information collected at the level of the nursing unit. This database was initiated by the American Nurses Association (ANA) and began in 1997 when the ANA selected the Midwest Research Institute and the University of Kansas School of Nursing to take on the task to develop and maintain the NDNQI. From 1997 to 2000 the ANA funded several studies to test selected indicators. Since then the database has grown tremendously in the number of indicators evaluated and in the number of participating hospitals.

Benefits
One of the biggest benefits of the National Database of Nursing Quality Indicators (NDNQI) comes from the comparisons generated from participating hospitals. In 1998 the NDNQI started accepting data from participating hospitals and then began to charge for data submission and the creation of comparison reports in 2001. Comparison information is grouped based on the patient and unit type. Quarterly reports provide information including national comparisons along with performance trends of the specific unit over the last eight quarters. Many hospitals utilize this information to assist with quality improvement, nursing recruitment and retention, patient

recruitment, research, and development of staff education topics. This information is also valuable to the participating hospital because it can be utilized to meet report requirements for different regulatory bodies or magnet designations.

<u>Nursing-sensitive indicators</u>
The nursing process, structure, and patient outcomes from nursing care are shown through the nursing-sensitive indicators. The nursing process indicators evaluate nursing assessment, interventions, and job satisfaction. The structure of nursing care is shown through the number of nursing staff members as well as the skill level, educational level, and any certifications of the nursing staff. Patient outcomes that are considered sensitive to nursing interventions include incidents such as skin breakdown, falls, or intravenous fluid infiltrates. The occurrence of these types of incidents can be directly correlated to quantity or quality of nursing care.

Basic level of nursing practice

There are two main levels of nursing practice within the psychiatric mental health field. There is the basic level of practice and then the advanced level of practice. Nurses that practice under the basic level belong to one of two subgroups. The first subgroup includes registered nurses that function in the role of a general staff nurse in a mental health facility, case managers, nurse managers, or other various nursing roles. The second subgroup includes the psychiatric-mental health nurse (RN-PMH), which is a baccalaureate prepared registered nurse that has practiced in the mental health field for at least two years. The functions of a nurse practicing at the basic level may include health promotion, education, intake admission screening and evaluation, case management, milieu therapy, promotion of self-care, psychobiologic interventions, counseling, crisis care, and rehabilitation.

Professional performance and development

All professional psychiatric nurses are expected to achieve and maintain competent nursing practice as identified by the standards of professional performance found in the Scope and Standards of Psychiatric-Mental Health Nursing by the American Nurses Association. The defined standards of practice include quality of care, performance appraisal, education, collegiality, ethics, collaboration, research, and resource utilization. The nurse is evaluated against each of these standards of care, with the achievement of becoming and remaining competent being each nurse's own professional responsibility.

Performance appraisals of the psychiatric mental health nurse

A performance appraisal is one in which the nurse evaluates their own psychiatric mental health nursing practice in regards to standards of practice, statutes, and regulations that are relevant to their field of practice. There are two types of performance appraisals: the administrative performance appraisal and the clinical performance appraisal. The administrative performance appraisal reviews the nurse's performance against role expectations. It should identify areas needing improvement and areas in which the nurse has achieved competency. The clinical performance appraisal provides guidance through clinical supervision with a mentor. The mentor will have greater clinical experience, skill, and education. The purpose of this relationship is to provide the nurse with a support mechanism. They can share clinical, developmental, and emotional information with their confidant in order to gain knowledge and grow within their field of practice. This appraisal reviews clinical care and also functions as a support role.

Advanced level of nursing practice

The advanced level of nursing practice within the psychiatric mental health field is the second level of practice. This registered nurse has a master's level degree and is licensed as an advanced registered nurse practitioner psychiatric-mental health (ARNP – PMH) and functions as a clinical specialist or a nurse practitioner. The ARNP-PMH is nationally certified as a psychiatric mental health specialist by the American Nurses Credentialing Center (ANCC). The advanced level of practice also includes nurses who have earned a doctorate in nursing (DNS, DNSc) or a doctorate of philosophy (PhD). Nurses functioning at this level can provide complete delivery of direct primary mental health services. They are able to diagnose, order, evaluate, or interpret diagnostic information. They are also able to conduct psychotherapy, pharmacotherapy, and monitor the patient's progress in regards to both types of intervention.

Continued learning process

Health care in general is rapidly changing each and every day. There are always new advances and information available for the nurse to continue to learn within their specific field of practice. The boundaries and practice of nursing is ever changing along with expectations of care. Nurses are expected to actively engage in seeking out ways to continue the learning process and keep up with the newest information. Examples of ways to do this can include: formal or continuing educational programs, independent learning, attending lectures, conferences or workshops, credentialing, or obtaining specialty certifications. Reading the latest journals or simply talking with peers are great ways to increase one's knowledge base.

Clinical supervision

Clinical supervision involves a learning process that provides the means for promoting positive change. There are four main forms of supervision. These include the dyadic, triadic, group, and peer review. The dyadic is a one-on-one relationship in which the supervisor and the individual meet face to face. The triadic is a relationship in which two nurses meet with the supervisor. The group setting is one in which more than two nurses meet with the supervisor. Peer review involves nurses meeting together without the involvement of supervision to perform evaluations of clinical practice. Each of these forms shares a common goal: to explore problems and strengths of the nurses being supervised.

APNA and ISPN

The American Psychiatric Nurses Association (APNA) is the largest psychiatric nursing organization that focuses upon the advancement of nursing practice along with continued improvements in cultural diversity, families, groups, and communities. The International Society of Psychiatric-Mental Health Nurses (ISPN) is composed of three specialty divisions that include the Association of Child and Adolescent Psychiatric Nurses, the International Society of Psychiatric Consultation Liaison Nurses, and the Society for Education and Research in Psychiatric-Mental Health Nursing. The main goal of the ISPN is to bring together all psychiatric-mental health nurses and to advance quality care available for both the individual and the family unit. Many of these organizations have annual meetings where newest information on the forefront of mental health nursing is presented. There are membership fees to join these associations.

Psychiatric mental health nursing organizations

Professional organizations provide nurses with the latest medical information, support meaningful legislation that encourages quality patient care through exceptional nursing care, and a body of leadership to help guide the future of nursing. One of the best known and largest nursing organizations is the American Nurses Association (ANA). The ANA provides support to the mental health nursing field through advocacy at the national and state levels and also through collaboration with other psychiatric-mental health nursing organizations. The American Psychiatric Nurses Association (APNA) and the International Society of Psychiatric-Mental Health Nurses (ISPN) are two other well respected large organizations that support the mental health field of nursing.

Presentations

Preparation
When preparing a presentation for peers, interdisciplinary members of the health care team, accreditation agencies, or anytime an individual will be speaking publicly, preparation is the most important part of a successful presentation. Many times the most difficult task of preparing a presentation is actually getting started. First, all the facts and information on the subject should be gathered and reviewed. Determine which information is the most important along with how much and what parts of the content should be presented. Try not to read the presentation. Use of visual aids as a guide with topic headings and subheadings can be a very effective tool to help prompt the speaker on the subject. When utilizing visual aids within the presentation, always practice and be informed about how to utilize the equipment.

Organization
Most presentations can be organized into three main sections. These sections include an introduction, body, and conclusion. The introduction should include the main purpose of the presentation and can include important statistics or facts. The body should include the main ideas and the conclusion should summarize all the information presented and can allow for questions and answers. Determine a format for the presentation by deciding upon a sequence. This section can be organized by simply stating a sequence of events, placing information into categories, stating problems and solutions, or providing contrasts and comparisons. Then decide if visual aids should be utilized and what type will most effectively present the information. Examples of visual aids include a flip chart, transparencies, and more commonly the use of an LCD projector. Visual aids can include words, pictures, graphs, or charts.

Omnibus Budget Reconciliation Act and the Nursing Home Reform Amendments

The Omnibus Budget Reconciliation Act of 1987 was amended in 1990 with Nursing Home Reform Amendments. These amendments establish guidelines for nursing facilities (e.g., long-term care facilities). The provisions include the following:
- There must be a complete physical and mental assessment of each patient on admission, annually, and with a change of condition.
- It is required that for every 24-hour period, a registered nurse must be on duty for at least one 8-hour shift.
- Nurses' aide training is mandated in addition to regular in-service and state registry of trained or qualified aides.
- Rehabilitative services must be available.

- A physician, a physician's assistant, or a nurse practitioner must visit once every 30 days for the first 3 months and then once every 90 days thereafter.
- Medicaid discrimination is outlawed.
- There is a requirement for independent monitoring of psychopharmacologic drugs.
- Patients' rights are recognized.
- Survey protocols to assess patient care and patient outcomes must be in place.
- There are state sanctions to enforce nursing home regulations.

Quality improvement or process improvement

Quality improvement or process improvement focus on the patient, program of care as a whole, and patient outcomes. The purpose of quality or process improvement is to create, implement, evaluate, and change or guide the improvement of care provided by the organization. Identified objectives include the following: efficient use of resources, ongoing improvement in customer satisfaction and patient outcomes, and adherence to professional and regulatory standards.   Nurses often participate in this process through the identification of problem areas that need improvement. Many times nurses are on the front line of providing patient care and are the experts at identifying problem areas. Nurses can also participate in data collection necessary to evaluate the current process or a newly implemented process.

Quality improvement of nursing care delivery

Scientific management theory and motivation theory
Two traditional organizational behavior theories are Frederick Taylor's scientific management theory (1917) and Elton Mayo's motivation theory (1933).
- Scientific management theory: Management's role was to plan and control, identifying tasks, assigning the best person to complete the tasks, and using both rewards and punishment as motivating forces. This theory focuses on outcomes rather than on individuals, and workers are often not motivated within this structure.
- Motivation theory: This theory requires that managers take a personal interest in the needs of workers. It was found that workers responded positively to changes in the working environment; they were motivated by increased managerial interest and involvement, team work, and improved communication between management and staff where workers were included in the decision-making process.

Performance improvement models
A number of different performance improvement models have been developed. Evaluating and applying these models are part of strategic management and quality health care. Often models are combined to meet specific needs. Planning and understanding how these models facilitate change are important for those in leadership positions because there must be cooperation and consensus across the organization for these models to be effective. The various models share some elements:
- These models focus on continuous improvement; are planned, systematic, and collaborative; and apply to the entire organization.
- These models share a common focus on identifying problems, collecting data, assessing current performance, instituting changes, assessing changes, developing teams, and using data.
- A model that is appropriate to the needs of the organization and its employees is most likely to be successful.

Continuous quality improvement

Continuous quality improvement (CQI) emphasizes the organization and the systems and processes within that organization rather than individuals. It recognizes internal customers (staff) and external customers (patients), using collected data to improve processes. CQI uses the scientific method of experimentation to meet needs and improve services, using various tools, such as brainstorming, storyboarding, and meetings. Core concepts include the following:

- Quality and success are meeting or exceeding internal and external customers' needs and expectations.
- Problems relate to processes, and variations in process lead to variations in results.
- Change can occur in small steps.
- Steps to CQI include the following:
- Forming a knowledgeable team
- Identifying and defining measures used to determine success
- Brainstorming strategies for change
- Planning, collecting, and using data as part of making decisions
- Testing changes and revising or refining them as needed

Total quality management
Total quality management (TQM) espouses a commitment to meeting the needs of customers at all levels within an organization. It promotes not only continuous improvement but also a dedication to quality. Outcomes include increased customer satisfaction, productivity, and profits through efficiency and cost reductions. To provide TQM, an organization must seek the following:

- Information regarding customer's needs and opinions
- Involvement of staff at all levels of decision-making, goal-setting, and problem-solving
- Commitment of management to empowering staff and being accountable through active leadership and participation
- Institution of teamwork with incentives and rewards for accomplishments
- The focus of TQM is on working together to identify and solve problems rather than assigning blame.

Research utilization
Research utilization requires critical thinking skills to evaluate insights gained from research and then applying them to practice; this must be an ongoing effort on the part of the clinical nurse specialist (CNS), who must stay current with new developments in his or her field of interest. Because much research is not disseminated widely, the CNS must actively seek new information from journals, society meetings, libraries, and the Internet, focusing on areas of interest or need. Research utilization varies widely; thus, staff must be educated so that all members adopt a similar approach to research utilization, applying that approach consistently and evaluating outcomes.

Integrating the results of data analysis
Integrating the results of data analysis is essential for identifying opportunities for performance improvement and developing practice guidelines. These data are used for long-term strategic planning on an ongoing basis. Integration of information includes the following:

- Identifying issues for tracking
- Reviewing patterns and trends to determine how they impact care
- Establishing action plans and desired outcomes based on the need for improvement
- Providing information to process improvement teams to facilitate change
- Evaluating systems and processes for follow-up

- Monitoring specific cases, criteria, critical pathways, and outcomes
- The integration of information can help with case management, decision-making about individual care, improvement of critical pathways related to clinical performance, staff performance evaluations, credentialing, and privileging.

Nurse's role in furthering new research

As health care providers it is each nurse's responsibility to observe patient outcomes and evaluate the effectiveness of treatments and interventions. Through this front-row seat research, ideas can be identified and developed. Descriptive and exploratory research can define the problem and influencing factors and a hypothesis can then be developed. Cause-and-effect relationships can then be tested in either natural or controlled environments. After a cause and effect relationship has been identified, specific interventions directed towards the resolution of a problem can then be tested through randomized controlled clinical trials. The nurse can participate in any or all of these different steps. They can contribute to the initial idea, collect data, monitor outcomes, or assist with ongoing reevaluation of the problem.

Purposes of documentation

Documentation is a form of communication that provides information about the patient and confirms that care was provided. Accurate, objective, and complete documentation of individual care is required by both accreditation and reimbursement agencies, including federal and state governments. The purposes of documentation include the following:
- Carrying out professional responsibility
- Establishing accountability
- Communicating among health professionals
- Educating staff
- Providing information for research
- Satisfying legal and practice standards
- Ensuring reimbursement

While documentation focuses on progress notes, there are many other aspects to charting. Physician's orders must be noted, medication administration must be documented on medication sheets, and vital signs must be graphed. Flow sheets must be checked off, filled out, or initialed. Admission assessments may involve primarily checklists or may require extensive documentation. The primary issue in malpractice cases is inaccurate or incomplete documentation. It is better to overdocument than underdocument, but the most effective documentation does neither.

Accuracy in documentation

Regardless of format, documentation should always include any change in a patient's condition, any treatments, medications or other interventions, patient responses, and any complaints of family or patient. Nurses should avoid subjective descriptions (especially negative terms, which could be used to establish bias in court), such as tired, angry, confused, bored, rude, happy, and euphoric. Instead, more objective descriptions, such as "Yawning 2–3 times a minute," should be used. Patients can be quoted directly, "I shouldn't have to wait for medication when I need it!" Charting should focus on nursing diagnoses. Nurses should update a patient's chart every 1–2 hours for routine care (e.g., bathing, walking), but medications and other interventions or changes in condition should be recorded immediately. A standardized vocabulary should be used for documentation, including lists of approved abbreviations and symbols. Abbreviations and symbols, especially, can pose serious problems in interpretation, so they should be used sparingly.

EMR

The electronic medical record (EMR) is a computerized patient record, which may be integrated with computerized physician/provider order entries and clinical decision support systems to improve individual care and reduce medical errors. Software applications vary considerably as standardization has not yet been implemented. When converting to a health care delivery system that uses EMR, there is a need for extensive training for all staff at all levels; all procedures that are currently paper-related must be modified and converted to a digital format. Standard terminology may need to be established or modified. Staff must be trained to input and retrieve information from the electronic system; safeguards must be built into the system to prevent violations of confidentiality. Information retrievable from the Internet must be encrypted. Computer screens must be outside the line of sight of visitors or unauthorized individuals, and retrieval of records must use secure PINS and passwords.

Practice guidelines

Practice guidelines provide strategies for delivery of care. These are developed to assist with decisions involving clinical interventions, to provide patients with valuable educational information, and to ensure effective treatments. The goals of practice guidelines include definitive documentation of preferred practices, provision of consistency of care, utilization of outcome based research, improved quality of care, increased staff productivity, and reduced health care costs. The most effective practice guidelines are based upon current clinical research information to determine the most effective treatments for specific disorders. These guidelines should be monitored and reevaluated frequently to ensure that they are based upon the latest and most accurate research information.

Limitations

While practice guidelines are important tools utilized to ensure quality patient care and outcomes, they can also have certain limitations. These guidelines may not always allow for patient variables that can affect outcomes. These variables include individual patient characteristics, the varying nature of the therapeutic relationship, treatment interventions, and the placebo effect. Practice guidelines are also often developed from the focus of a single discipline and may not incorporate a multidisciplinary view. They can also be very rigid and not allow for flexibility to meet the needs of each individual patient.

Development of evidence based practice

The development of evidence based practice involves a series of steps. The first step is to determine the clinical question that needs to be answered. This question needs to be very specific and determined by the identification of a patient problem, existing nursing interventions, and the expected patient outcome. The second step in this process is to locate the evidence. This evidence can be found from various sources including the internet, journals, or various medical libraries. The evidence then needs to be critically evaluated for reliability and realistic application to the specific named question. One of the most reliable forms of information is a meta-analysis of randomized controlled trials (RCT). After the evidence has been evaluated, it should then be put into practice. The use of practice guidelines is one of the best ways to utilize this information. The final step is to evaluate the patient outcomes based upon the evidence based care. This information is gathered through outcome measurement and continued evaluation.

Nursing Code of Ethics

The American Nurses Association developed the Nursing Code of Ethics. There are nine provisions, which are listed below:

- The nurse treats all patients with respect and consideration, regardless of social circumstances or health condition.
- The nurse's primary commitment is to the patient, regardless of conflicts that may arise.
- The nurse promotes and advocates for the patients' health, safety, and rights, maintaining privacy and confidentiality and protecting them from questionable practices or care.
- The nurse is responsible for his or her own care practices and determines appropriate delegation of care.
- The nurse must retain respect for him- or herself and his or her integrity and competence.
- The nurse ensures that the health care environment is conducive to providing good health care and is consistent with professional and ethical values.
- The nurse participates in education and knowledge development to advance the profession.
- The nurse collaborates with others to promote efforts to meet health needs.
- The nursing profession articulates values and promotes and maintains the integrity of the profession.

Ethical and standards of care violations

The nurse has an obligation to report ethical and standards of care violations and to intervene to ensure the safety of the patient. This obligation is outlined by state boards of nursing, professional organizations, and accrediting agencies. The nurse must report suspected or observed diversion of drugs; any type of abuse (e.g., physical, emotional, sexual, financial); falsification of patient records; neglect of patients; narcotic offenses; and arrests, indictments, or convictions for criminal offenses. Each facility should have policies in place for reporting, but the usual procedure is to report violations to the immediate supervisor and file an incident report; however, the nurse can file a complaint directly with the board of nursing, especially if the matter is serious. The written report is essential in the event that the nurse experiences reprisals. After filing a report, the nurse should follow up to determine if action has been taken. With ethical dilemmas, a report may be made to the bioethics committee. Violations may result in disciplinary action, mentoring, or loss of a license.

Ethical dilemmas

Ethics is the study of morals and encompasses concepts of right and wrong. When dealing with ethical dilemmas, one must consider not only what people should do but also what they actually do. Ethical issues can be difficult to assess because of personal bias, which is one of the reasons that sharing concerns with other internal sources, such as an ethics committee, and reaching consensus is so valuable. Issues of concern might include options for care, refusal of care, rights to privacy, adequate relief of suffering, and the right to self-determination. Internal sources, such as an ethics committee, are given the responsibility to make decisions on ethical issues. Risk management can provide guidance related to personal and institutional liability. External agencies, such as the public health department, may also be consulted on ethical dilemmas.

Ethical decision-making

It is important for nurses to avoid making decisions solely based on their beliefs that they know what is best for individuals. In 1998, P. S. Chally and L. Loriz developed a model for ethical decision-making for nurses to use when faced with ethical dilemmas or choices (Chally PS, Loriz L. Decision making in practice. *Am J Nurs*. 98(6),17–20, 1998). Steps to ethical decision-making include the following:

- Clarifying the extent/type of dilemma and who is ultimately responsible for making the decision
- Obtaining more data, including information about legal issues, such as the obligation to report
- Considering alternative solutions
- Arriving at a decision after considering risks and benefits and discussing it with the individual
- Acting on the decision and using collaboration as needed
- Assessing the outcomes of the decision to determine if the chosen action was effective

Patient rights

Patient's bill of rights

Due to the nature of their illness, many mentally ill patients received very poor care in the past. Their illnesses and behaviors were not well understood. Care providers for patients with mental disorders have to balance patient and staff safety concerns along with appropriate patient treatments and ethical and legal rights. To address the mistreatment of many of these patients, certain laws have been enacted. Many hospitals and outpatient treatment facilities utilize a patient's bill of rights. These rights are provided to the patient upon admission and are read or explained to them. In 1980, the Mental Health Systems Act was passed into law and provides certain universal rights for mental health patients. In 1973, the American Hospital Association also developed a Patient's Bill of Rights, which is utilized by many of the treatment facilities in the United States.

Communication with others outside the hospital and the right to keep personal effects

When a patient is admitted into an inpatient facility or during their time at an outpatient facility they have certain rights. One of these rights is the right to communicate with others outside the hospital. The patient is allowed to have visits from parents, friends, and family. They may also have private telephone conversations and send unread sealed mail. There may be specific visitation or phone usage times designated by the treatment facility. However, if the patient may be harmed or intends to harm someone else, their contact may be limited by the facility. The right to keep personal effects allows the patient to bring their own clothes and certain personal items into the facility. Items that may be dangerous to the patient or others will be confiscated and held by the facility.

Right to education and habeas corpus

The United States Constitution guarantees the right to education to everyone. Many times parents of intellectually disabled children will seek to provide for their education. All states are required to provide education to all citizens. Habeas corpus is a constitutional right that provides for the quick release of any individual that claims to be detained against their will or illegally. This right is particularly important to those patients admitted involuntarily. They may file a legal writ based on the grounds that they are sane and eligible for discharge. This is a court hearing and will hear the reasons why the person was committed from those who requested the action. The patient will be discharged if they are found to be sane.

Right to enter into a contractual relationship and the issue of mental incompetence

As long as a patient is capable of understanding the nature of a contract and their judgment is not impaired, the court of law will uphold any contracts signed by a psychiatric patient. When a patient is considered incompetent they are considered incapable of making contractual agreements or tending to their own personal affairs. To prove an individual is incompetent in a court of law the person must have a diagnosed mental disorder that causes impaired judgment and renders the individual incapable of making appropriate decisions concerning their personal affairs. If an individual is declared incompetent, the court of law will appoint a guardian to manage their affairs. If found incompetent, an individual also cannot get married, vote, drive, or sign contracts.

Right to informed consent

Each patient has the right to informed consent concerning any recommended treatments. The patient must be given information about the treatment including any possible complications or risks. Additional information should include their diagnosis, purpose of the treatment, alternative options, and the expected outcome. In order for a patient to give informed consent for their treatments they must be considered competent. The competent patient should be able to communicate their choices, comprehend important relevant information, understand the situation and its consequences, and be able to logically understand the risks versus benefits of the treatment.

Right to privacy

The right to privacy allows the patient to keep certain information confidential. Confidentiality protects the patient's information from others unless they are authorized to see it by the patient. In April 2003, the Health Insurance Portability and Accountability Act (HIPAA) was passed to provide patients with increased availability to their own medical information and how it is utilized and disclosed. Information is only shared with other members of the health care team who are directly involved in patient care. There are certain situations when the patient's information can be released without their consent. These usually involve court proceedings, emergency situations, or actions taken to protect another party.

> ➢ **Review Video:** Confidentiality
> Visit *mometrix.com/academy* and enter *Code:* **250384**

Right to treatment in the least restrictive setting

The right to treatment in the least restrictive setting addresses the needs of the patient and seeks to maintain the highest degree of personal dignity, autonomy, and freedom. This applies to the right of the patient not to be committed to an inpatient facility if they can be successfully treated in an outpatient setting. The use of seclusion and restraints is also a concern when utilizing the least restrictive setting. These two options should only be utilized in extreme circumstances and documentation should indicate the rationale for their utilization, alternative methods attempted, patient behavior while restrained or in seclusion, nursing interventions, and continuous monitoring and evaluation of the patient.

Right to treatment and the right to refuse treatment

The right to treatment applies to involuntarily admitted patients and only requires adequate minimal treatments. It does not require a range of treatment options or ensure the best treatments. The court of law has identified three criteria concerning adequate treatment. These criteria include the following: provision of a humane physical and psychological environment, sufficient numbers of qualified staff to provide care, and implementation of individualized treatment plans. In contrast, the right to refuse treatment involves the right to refuse involuntary admission to a treatment facility. The belief behind this right states that involuntary hospitalization goes against the basic rights of freedom of thought and the right to control one's own life and actions as long as they do not impact the rights of other people.

Forcing medications as coerced treatment

Many times patients that are suffering from a mental illness may refuse treatment with medications. These patients may be suffering from delirium, dementia, or psychosis. Patients who are admitted on a voluntary basis and are not violent towards themselves or others can refuse any treatment or medication. However, with patients that have been committed, there are certain criteria that can justify coerced treatment. These criteria include the following: the patient is dangerous to themselves or others, those administering treatment truly believe that the treatment has a good chance of helping the patient, and the patient has been determined to be incompetent. Many times a positive therapeutic relationship between the nurse and the patient can help avoid the refusal of treatments.

Patient Self-Determination Act

The Patient Self-Determination Act (1990), an amendment to the Omnibus Budget Reconciliation Act, allows a mental health patient to develop an advance psychiatric directive (APD) during a period when a professional mental health care provider certifies the person is of sound mind. The APD allows the patient to determine in advance the types of treatment that are acceptable and those that are not. The patient can also designate another person, such as a family member, to make decisions if the patient is unable to do so. State regulations regarding APDs vary somewhat. The APD is particularly valuable to those who have severe, chronic, psychiatric illnesses, such as schizophrenia, and who may face involuntary commitment. A patient may outline preferences regarding specific treatments and interventions, such as medications, seclusion, restraint, and electroshock therapy.

Confidentiality

The health care provider is under an ethical obligation to protect confidential information from being shared with others. Information exchanged between the patient and the healthcare provider is confidential. However, the patient may give permission for this information to be shared with others. Mental health providers discuss highly personal and vitally important information with their patients. Laws have been enacted to protect confidentiality. Information may concern other people as well as the patient themselves. Many of the patients must feel secure in the confidentiality of their information before they will share this information and seek the help they need. A person's location, such as admission to any treatment facility, is considered under the umbrella of confidentiality.

Sharing patient information

Patient information may need to be shared with other team members. These team members are only those involved with direct patient care and may include health care consults, other staff members caring for the patient, health care students and faculty, or supervisory staff. These team members need the patient information to be able to provide care for the patient. The patient also has the right to share their personal information with anyone they choose. There may also be other situations in which information may need to be shared such as criminal proceedings, child abuse or custody hearings, when acting in the patient's best interests during emergencies, court-ordered evaluations, acting to protect third parties, or in reports required by state law, such as CDC reportable diseases or gunshot wounds.

Protecting a third party from harm

Many laws are in place to protect a person's confidentiality. However, if a person intends to harm someone else, then the information must be shared to protect the other person. This responsibility requires the health care provider to assess the reality of the threat against another person, identify the person at risk, and begin an action to prevent the harmful act. The health care provider must determine if the patient is dangerous to others and whether or not it is due to serious mental illness. The provider must also attempt to determine how soon the patient could harm someone else. The patient's privacy may still be able to be protected. However, the possible threat of harm should be shared.

HIPAA

The Health Insurance Portability and Accountability Act (HIPAA) went into effect in 2003. This act came about in part because of the ease of access to patient information through computer databases. Due to the increased availability of patient information by so many other people, the patient's privacy was in need of increased protection. HIPAA increased the patient's control over their health care information. HIPAA determined four rights concerning patient information:
- The patient must be educated about HIPAA
- The patient must have access to their medical records.
- The patient may request that information they object to be changed or corrected.
- The patient's permission must be obtained before any information is shared.

Confidentiality and privacy

Confidentiality is the ethical obligation of the health care provider to keep information exchanged with the patient from being shared with others. A patient's privacy involves keeping secret certain aspects of their personal life. There can be situations in which privacy is broken, but confidentiality is not. Many of the patient's staying in inpatient treatment facilities may have their privacy broken by observances of staff members, but if this information is not shared, then confidentiality remains intact. Confidentiality helps to build trust between the patient and provider. The provider is bound both morally and ethically to protect the information of the patient.

Risk management

Many treatment facilities will have a department that deals with risk management. A risk is the possibility that something bad could happen. Risk managers attempt to decrease the probability of negative patient outcomes due to the patient care they received. Nurses that work in this area identify risk factors that could not only negatively affect the individual patient, but could cause system wide problems. These factors can be identified through audits and evaluation of complaints and occurrence reports. They seek to develop corrective actions and strategies to reduce patient risk and liability issues.

Resource utilization

Resource utilization refers to the consideration of all factors related to the planning and delivery of quality patient care. These factors may include patient safety, treatment effectiveness, and cost of care. The patient should receive mental health care that meets all of the factors. The care should be safe, effective and affordable for each individual patient. Treatment decisions should take into consideration rising health care costs and how to maximize the use of certain resources while continuing to provide quality patient care. The goal of resource utilization is to provide quality, cost effective care while utilizing the best qualified and appropriate resources.

Scope of specialty practice

The scope of specialty practice is regulated by each state's board of nursing, usually according to educational preparation; in most cases clinical nurse specialists (CNSs) are categorized as advanced practice nurses, and there is little difference in the responsibilities given to the CNS and those given to the nurse practitioner. However the psychiatric and mental health CNS must practice within the limits of the state regulations, personal competency level, and professional ethical standards. The role of the CNS is to promote mental health through the nursing process and to provide patient-centered nursing care and evaluation of outcomes in a variety of settings. The CNS should promote wellness, prevention, and treatment to allow the mental health patient to function as independently as possible.

Violations of legal and regulatory requirements

Depending on the seriousness of the issue, the nurse may report violations of legal and regulatory requirements to an immediate supervisor, according to established protocol, or directly to a regulatory agency. In almost all cases, regulatory agencies, such as the Occupational Safety and Health Administration, provide a way (e.g., online, fax, mail, telephone) to file a confidential complaint and protect the person from reprisals, such as firing or demotion. Some issues have a timeline, so reports should be completed immediately when the nurse becomes aware of violations. Additionally, each state has regulatory boards that are responsible for investigating violations of legal and regulatory standards, and these regulatory boards should investigate and take action after a complaint is filed. There are specific federal and state regulations that cover breaches of confidentiality of health information, which require health care professionals, Health and Human Services (if more than 500 patients are involved), and the media to be notified.

Problems affecting quality of care and patient safety

Each medical facility should have an established policy that identifies problems, such as quality variances, sentinel events, and infections, which pose a risk to the quality of care and patient safety. These problems should prompt a case review and an analysis. The policy should clearly define problems (e.g., sentinel events) and outline the processes for reporting, recording, and managing the problems as well as appropriate preventive methods. Depending on the type of event, the nurse who identifies a problem reports to the physician, a supervisor, or another appropriate department, such as infection control or a regulatory agency. Suicides are the second most common sentinel event reported to the Joint Commission. "Never events," that is, those that should never happen in a medical care setting (e.g., suicide, accidental death, medication error), should always be reported, according to established protocol.

Sentinel events

Sentinel events are defined by the Joint Commission as a death or serious physical injury that is unexpected. This death or injury could be related to many things, including surgery on the wrong body part, suicide, or infection. An infection is considered a sentinel event if it is determined that the death or injury would not have occurred without the infection. Each case must be dealt with individually, and if defined as sentinel, a root-cause analysis, which collects evidence to identify contributions to the problem, must be done. Once a root cause has been determined, an action plan that identifies all the different elements that contributed to the problem is instituted. The theory is that finding the root cause can eliminate the problem rather than just treating it. Thus, finding the source of an infection is more important than simply administering an antibiotic to treat the infection.

Epidemiologically significant organisms

Epidemiologically significant organisms are those with the potential to cause death, disease, or serious injury. Some organisms are considered significant because they are invasive and cause outbreaks but also are often resistant to antimicrobials, making control difficult. When epidemiologically significant organisms are identified, usually through active surveillance or cultures, enhanced infection control may be needed to control the spread of infection. Microorganisms that are significant include vancomycin-resistant *enterococci*, *Clostridium difficile*, methicillin-resistant *Staphylococcus aureus,* as well as others that can be transmitted directly or indirectly. Antibiotic resistance is increasing among gram-negative bacilli such as *Klebsiella pneumoniae, Pseudomonas aeruginosa,* and *Enterobacter* spp. Significant organisms may vary from one department to another; even though some organisms might be fatal to neonates but pose little threat to adults, health care facilities must be viewed as a single unit because of the ease with which infections can spread and become more virulent.

Assessment of patient exposure to communicable disease

Patient exposure to communicable disease can be difficult to assess as the person may not be aware of exposure or may be reluctant to discuss it because of privacy issues. Doing a careful and thorough history and physical assessment can provide information that suggests exposure. Questioning patients about symptoms rather than diseases may elicit more information: "Have you had contact with anyone with a rash?" or "Have you experienced night sweats?" Exposure to a communicable disease can occur inside and outside of the hospital. Exposure to communicable disease can be endogenous (self-infection) or exogenous (cross-infection). Endogenous infections, for example, can result from the normal body flora or an area of infection (e.g., a boil) contaminating a surgical wound. Exogenous infections can occur by contact with someone who is infected, such as another patient or staff member, or by airborne particles. Both types of infection occur in the hospital.

Coordination of intra- and interdisciplinary teams

There are a number of skills that are needed to lead and facilitate coordination of intra- and interdisciplinary teams for patient care, which are listed below:
- Communicating openly is essential with all members encouraged to participate as valued members of a cooperative team.
- It is important to avoid interrupting or interpreting the point another is trying to make to allow a free flow of ideas.
- It is important to avoid jumping to conclusions, which can effectively shut off communication.
- Active listening requires that health care professions pay attention and ask questions for clarification rather than challenging the ideas of other health care professionals.
- Respecting the opinions and ideas of others, even when they are opposed to one's own, is absolutely essential.

- Reacting and responding to facts rather than feelings allows one to avoid angry confrontations or diffuse anger.
- Clarifying information or opinions stated can help avoid misunderstandings.
- Keeping unsolicited advice out of the conversation shows respect for other professionals, allowing them to solicit advice without feeling pressured.

Interdisciplinary collaboration

Interdisciplinary collaboration is absolutely critical to nursing practice if the needs and best interests of the patients and their families are central. Interdisciplinary practice begins with the nurse and physician but extends to pharmacists, social workers, occupational and physical therapists, nutritionists, and a wide range of allied health care providers, all of whom cooperate in diagnosis and treatment; however, state regulations determine to some degree how much autonomy a nurse can have in diagnosing and treating patients. While nurses have increasingly gained more legal rights, they are also dependent on collaboration with others for their expertise and for referrals if the patient's needs extend beyond the nurse's ability to provide assistance. Additionally, the prescriptive ability of nurses varies from state to state, with some states requiring direct supervision by physicians while others require other types of supervisory arrangements.

Interdisciplinary communication and documentation

Psychiatric patients usually have many different people involved in providing their care. Collaboration between the many different disciplines is crucial in providing a positive patient outcome. These different disciplines can include family members, nurses, medical doctors, psychiatrists, psychologists, social workers, case workers, and other therapists or counselors. Therefore interdisciplinary communication is vital in assuring positive patient outcomes. Because each member of this team usually functions independently of the other, most facilities have an organized method to provide regular communication between each discipline.

Problems with utilizing an interdisciplinary approach

Many times the collaborative process between the different disciplines involved in caring for the psychiatric patient does not proceed without some difficulties. Many times the roles and functions of the team members may overlap. This can lead to confusion of exactly what each team member is to contribute to the patient outcome. For the collaborative process to work smoothly, team members should agree upon a common philosophy, respect each other's input, clearly define each member's role and responsibility, specify a hierarchy of decision making, and communicate on a regular basis.

Nurse's role as patient advocate

Patient advocacy has long been a role of the nurse. Nurses are there to care for inpatients 24 hours a day 7 days a week. They are there to watch over and protect the well-being of each patient. As a patient advocate, nurses often provide simple easily understandable education. This education encompasses many complex medical terms and explanations that are put into a language that the average person can easily understand. This teaching can include medications, procedures, treatments, and goals of therapy. Along with inpatient advocacy, community and public health are areas that the nurse can expand into to provide valuable education. By educating a group or entire community, the nurse can effect real change and assist others to seek help and recognize symptoms of problems that they normally would not have realized.

- 99 -

Healthy People 2020 agenda

Healthy People 2020 was initiated by the Department of Health and Human Services in January 2010 to challenge the nation to improve health promotion and disease prevention. This agenda calls on individuals, professionals, and entire communities to take specific steps to promote good health for everyone during the first decade of this century. It is composed of 42 specific areas. Each of these areas represents a public health issue with targeted improvements by the year 2020. Some examples of the areas of quality health care for which everyone should have access to include cancer, diabetes, heart disease and stroke, substance abuse, mental health, oral health, and family planning. This agenda also includes specific leading health indicators. These indicators are made up of objectives intended to aid all people in the understanding of health promotion and disease prevention.

Mental health is one of the leading health indicators with specific objectives identified by the Healthy People 2020 agenda. Some of these objectives include the following goals: a reduction in the overall suicide rate and adolescent suicide attempts; reduction of the mentally ill homeless population; increased employment rates for the mentally ill; decreased relapse rates for anorexia and bulimia nervosa; increased rates of mental health screening in primary care and juvenile justice facilities; increased rates of treatment for children and adults suffering from mental illness; increased rates of treatment for both substance abuse and mental illness when they occur together; increased tracking of patient satisfaction concerning mental health services; increased number of states and territories with an operational mental health plan that addresses cultural competence; and increased number of plans that address crisis intervention, ongoing screening, and treatment services available for the elderly population.

Nurse's own self-awareness

To be able to assist others with their mental health needs, it is vitally important that the nurse be aware of their own personal qualities, beliefs, and growth potential. The nurse needs to have some sense of self and understand their own motivations and limitations. They must be able to deal with the broad range of emotions they may feel when assisting patients with their mental health needs. Self-awareness should be examined through philosophical, psychological, physical, and environmental factors. The nurse needs to be open to exploring their own thoughts, emotions, and values. By having a better sense of self, the nurse should be able to become more objective when dealing with patient situations that may conflict with his or her own personal beliefs.

Practice Test

Practice Questions

1. A rape victim with multiple injuries has been brought to the emergency department for evaluation and treatment. The first thing that the psychiatric and mental health nurse should communicate is:
   - a. "I'm so sorry this happened to you."
   - b. "You are safe here. No one can hurt you."
   - c. "This was not your fault."
   - d. "I'm thankful you survived this attack."

2. A patient has signed the consent form for electroconvulsive therapy under pressure from her spouse but confides in the psychiatric and mental health nurse that she does not want the treatment and is terrified but is afraid to stand up to her spouse. The psychiatric and mental health nurse should:
   - a. Ask the patient if she wants to rescind the consent form.
   - b. Tell the patient that she must tell her spouse she does not want the treatment.
   - c. Tell the patient she must go through with the treatment since she signed the consent.
   - d. Notify the physician of the patient's feelings about the treatment.

3. A patient was able to slowly read aloud an information sheet but when asked to state what she had read in her own words was unable to do so. The most likely reason is:
   - a. low self-esteem.
   - b. poor hearing.
   - c. low health literacy.
   - d. anxiety.

4. A patient who has had repeated arrests for driving under the influence of alcohol refuses to admit that he has a drinking problem and states that the police have targeted him unfairly. The ego defense mechanism that the patient is using is:
   - a. denial.
   - b. reaction formation.
   - c. regression.
   - d. undoing.

5. A patient with schizophrenia has delusions and believes that his family members cannot be trusted. According to Maslow's hierarchy of needs, the patient's delusions are interfering with development at the level of:
   - a. physiological needs.
   - b. love/belonging needs.
   - c. safety needs.
   - d. self-esteem needs.

6. A patient states that, on the advice of a friend, he has been treating his anxiety with large doses of kava in addition to the amitriptyline that was prescribed for depression, but he has been feeling excessively fatigued and has noted dark urine. Which diagnostic test or tests are indicated?
    a. Renal function tests
    b. CBC
    c. Urinalysis
    d. Liver function tests

7. According to Erikson's stages of psychosocial development, which of the following best characterizes the developmental task of adulthood and the generativity vs. stagnation stage?
    a. Achieving self-confidence by performing successfully and gaining recognition from peers
    b. Developing a sense of positive self worth from reviewing the events of life
    c. Achieving the personal life goals that the person had formulated
    d. Making a commitment to another person as part of a long-term relationship

8. The International Society of Psychiatric-Mental Health Nurses (ISPN) contains how many divisions representing different nursing specialty areas?
    a. Two
    b. Four
    c. Six
    d. Eight

9. When utilizing AHRQ's *You Can Quit Smoking* guide to help a patient quit smoking, the first step of "Getting Ready" includes:
    a. Talking with the physician about nicotine medication.
    b. Telling friends and family members about quitting.
    c. Getting group counseling.
    d. Setting a date to quit, cold turkey.

10. An elderly patient scored 18 out of a possible maximum score of 30 on the Mini-Mental State Examination (MMSE). This score usually indicates:
    a. severe cognitive impairment.
    b. mild cognitive impairment.
    c. moderate cognitive impairment.
    d. normal cognition.

11. The psychiatric and mental health nurse needs to complete a history and physical examination on a patient who is extremely depressed and suicidal. The best approach is to:
    a. Delay the history and physical exam until the patient is stabilized.
    b. Conduct the baseline physical examination but delay the history taking.
    c. Obtain the history from a family member and conduct the physical exam.
    d. Conduct the history and physical in a supportive manner.

12. Piaget's theory of cognitive development in children applies to adults in relation to concepts about:
    a. readiness to learn.
    b. self-efficacy.
    c. self-determination.
    d. intelligence.

13. When conducting the brief mental status evaluation as part of the clinical interview, which of the following is an appropriate activity to evaluate the patient's ability to concentrate?
   a. List three objects and ask the patient to repeat the list immediately and again in a few minutes.
   b. Ask the patient to spell the word "world" in reverse.
   c. Ask the patient to carry out a two- to three-step task.
   d. Ask the patient what "a stitch in time saves nine" means.

14. Which of the following is a developmental milestone that usually occurs during adolescence (12 to 18 years)?
   a. Understanding abstract concepts.
   b. Comprehending and carrying out multiple directions in sequence.
   c. Understanding concepts of size and time.
   d. Enjoying doing things without assistance.

15. To reduce anxiety, the patient's plan of care calls for the patient to practice mindfulness meditation in order to detect symptoms before they become problematic. This is a technique used in:
   a. behavioral therapy.
   b. psychoanalytic therapy.
   c. cognitive therapy.
   d. cognitive behavioral therapy.

16. Which of the following is probably an example of normal cognitive changes associated with aging in an 85-year-old patient?
   a. A patient has forgotten how to use the stove to cook.
   b. A patient has forgotten attending a birthday party.
   c. A patient has forgotten which bank holds his savings account.
   d. A patient has forgotten to keep an appointment with the doctor.

17. When utilizing the HEEADSSS method to interview an adolescent, the three *Ss* refer to:
   a. Sexuality/Support/Secrets.
   b. Sexuality/Suicide/Safety.
   c. Suicide/Socialization/Shelter.
   d. Sexuality/Support/Suicide.

18. When using the reflective method during an interview, the best response to a patient's statement that his pain "moves around" is:
   a. "What do you mean?"
   b. "Where does it move around?"
   c. "Moves around?"
   d. "Could you be more specific?"

19. When admitting a new patient and reconciling medications, the psychiatric and mental health nurse finds one list of medications on a previous hospital record, another on the physician's notes, and a third provided by the patient. The first step is to:
   a. Compare all three lists.
   b. Ask the patient which list is correct.
   c. Ask the patient to prepare a new list.
   d. Utilize the latest list.

20. When completing the physical examination of a patient complaining of chest pain, the psychiatric and mental health nurse asks the patient where the chest pain is and the patient runs an index finger up and down the sternum (neck to epigastrium). This suggests that the pain is related to:
    a. angina.
    b. gastritis.
    c. heartburn.
    d. pleurisy.

21. A patient with bipolar disorder has been maintained on lithium with no problem for three years but develops sudden onset of nausea, vomiting, diarrhea, and generalized myopathy. The patient's lithium level is 1.8 mEq/L, which suggests:
    a. non-lithium-related symptoms.
    b. severe lithium toxicity.
    c. moderate lithium toxicity.
    d. mild lithium toxicity.

22. When planning a group discussion with patients about alcohol prevention, an important consideration when forming the group is that:
    a. The group members be diverse in levels of health literacy and conditions.
    b. The group members have similar levels of health literacy and conditions.
    c. The group members be chosen at random.
    d. The group members are all the same gender.

23. A 60-year-old female patient has been treated for depression with an SSRI for four months but reports no improvement in feelings of depression. The patient reports weight gain, lethargy, and feeling constantly "chilled." The patient probably needs:
    a. an increased dosage of medication.
    b. thyroid function tests.
    c. a change to a different medication.
    d. renal function tests.

24. A 78-year-old female patient has been alert and oriented but has sudden onset of confusion. She has no physical complaints but the psychiatric and mental health nurse finds a low-grade elevation of temperature on examination, leading the psychiatric and mental health nurse to suspect:
    a. a respiratory tract infection.
    b. onset of influenza.
    c. dehydration and malnutrition.
    d. a urinary tract infection.

25. Relapse prevention is part of the patient's individualized education plan on discharge. The statement that suggests the patient has made a realistic plan to prevent relapse is:
    a. "I know I have to stop taking drugs."
    b. "Don't worry. I've learned my lesson."
    c. "I will call my sponsor if I feel like using again."
    d. "My family will make sure I don't relapse."

26. Which of the following is considered a "positive" symptom of schizophrenia?
    a. Flat affect
    b. Disorganized speech
    c. Poor eye contact
    d. Impaired hygiene

27. A patient who believes that other people are constantly talking about him or laughing at him is likely experiencing delusions of:
    a. persecution.
    b. grandeur.
    c. reference.
    d. control.

28. A patient with anxiety disorder wants to utilize complementary therapy as an adjunct to anti-anxiety medications. The complementary therapy that is likely to be the most effective in providing relief from anxiety is:
    a. imagery/self-relaxation.
    b. acupuncture.
    c. massage.
    d. aromatherapy.

29. A patient frequently responds in rhymes, such as "The food is hot. I am hot and shot. The pot has been bought." This is an example of:
    a. word salad.
    b. clang associations.
    c. neologisms.
    d. associative looseness.

30. A male patient who is very short in stature has abused steroids in an attempt to build muscle mass. He excels in martial arts and he is very aggressive with other males. This behavior most likely reflects the ego defense mechanism of:
    a. identification.
    b. repression.
    c. introjection.
    d. compensation.

31. A patient exhibits disturbed thought processes and delusional thinking, insisting his room is "bugged by the CIA." The most appropriate response to the patient is:
    a. "That's not true. The CIA has no access to this facility."
    b. "OK, let's see if we can find the bug and remove it."
    c. "I understand you believe your room is bugged, but I don't believe it's possible."
    d. "Remember what you learned about hallucinations and delusions not being real."

32. A patient at risk for self-directed violence tells the psychiatric and mental health nurse that she wants to die and has nothing to live for. The most appropriate response is:
    a. "Do you have a suicide plan?"
    b. "Your family loves you very much."
    c. "You will feel better when the medication starts to work."
    d. "I'm so sorry to hear that, but I can help you."

33. A patient admitted to the psychiatric unit is withdrawn and fearful of others, staying in his room and remaining preoccupied with his own thoughts. The patient states he feels rejected by others. The most appropriate nursing diagnosis is:
   a. Powerlessness.
   b. Low self-esteem.
   c. Disturbed thought processes.
   d. Social isolation.

34. Which of the following medications is most likely to trigger a psychotic or manic response?
   a. Anticonvulsants
   b. Corticosteroids
   c. Antidepressants
   d. Opioids

35. The most common co-morbid condition in adolescents with bipolar disorder is:
   a. juvenile arthritis.
   b. lupus erythematosus.
   c. ADHD.
   d. dyslexia.

36. A patient experiences a sudden and severe panic attack and is almost paralyzed with fear, believing her life is in danger. In addition to providing an anti-anxiety medication, the most appropriate response for the psychiatric and mental health nurse is to:
   a. Leave the patient alone in a quiet space to recover.
   b. Ask the patient what would help relieve her anxiety.
   c. Stay with the patient and offer reassurance of safety.
   d. Remind the patient that her fears are not real.

37. The psychiatric and mental health nurse had developed a good relationship with a patient with borderline personality disorder, but the nurse took time off to deal with a family matter and when returning found the patient angry and resentful and blaming the nurse for her problems. This is an example of:
   a. manipulation.
   b. splitting.
   c. clinging/distancing.
   d. self-destructiveness.

38. A patient with bipolar disorder is extremely manipulative and often behaves in a sexually provocative and inappropriate manner with staff members and other patients. The most appropriate method(s) of dealing with this inappropriate behavior is to:
   a. Utilize positive reinforcement and negative consequences.
   b. Use chemical restraints to control inappropriate behavior.
   c. Refer the matter to the patient's psychiatrist for guidance.
   d. Isolate the patient from other patients until behavior improves.

39. A 16-year-old patient with anorexia nervosa weighs 76 pounds, is severely emaciated and malnourished, and has developed cardiac dysrhythmias. Nutrition is critical, but the patient refuses to eat any food. The most appropriate response for the psychiatric and mental health nurse is:
    a. "You will die if you don't eat."
    b. "You will be fed by nasogastric tube if you don't eat."
    c. "We can't help you if you don't help yourself."
    d. "I can't force you to eat." ~

40. A "state of optimum anxiety" refers to:
    a. readiness for learning.
    b. psychological well-being.
    c. readiness for therapy.
    d. response to treatment.

41. Patients being discharged from the psychiatric unit are referred to the outpatient Wellness Recovery Action Plan (WRAP) for group intervention. The primary focus of this program is to help patients to:
    a. Avoid relapses and rehospitalization.
    b. Avoid substance abuse.
    c. Identify needs for services.
    d. Identify personal wellness tools.

42. A patient with a long history of schizophrenia and alcohol and drug addiction with repeated institutionalizations is stabilized after the current hospitalization and is ready for discharge. Which of the following community resource referrals is most likely to be effective?
    a. Community Mental Health Center
    b. Psychiatric home health care
    c. Assertive Community Treatment (ACT)
    d. Partial hospitalization program

43. An Asian-American adolescent is to be discharged from a psychiatric unit after a psychotic episode, but the parents, who are immigrants from China, are adamant that the patient cannot receive any outpatient treatment or follow-up care, stating that his illness was caused by an "infection." The probable reason for this is:
    a. They are unfamiliar with Western treatment for mental illness.
    b. They have poor language skills and misunderstand the diagnosis.
    c. They have very low health literacy.
    d. They are ashamed their child has a psychiatric condition.

44. A patient has been classified as having a mild intellectual disability (IQ 60). Based on this, the psychiatric and mental health nurse expects that the patient is capable of:
    a. Achieving academic skills to a sixth-grade level.
    b. Achieving academic skills to a second-grade level.
    c. Learning through systematic habit forming.
    d. Responding to minimal training in self-help.

45. Which of the following is an example of a secondary health preventive measure?
   a. A public service campaign to educate the population about depression.
   b. A program to treat depression and prevent suicide.
   c. A screening event for all patients over age 55 with the Geriatric Depression Scale.
   d. A support group for patients with depression.

46. A patient in the emergency department with multiple injuries (bruises, split lip, facial laceration, head contusion) reports that her boyfriend got high on amphetamines and alcohol and beat her, so she drove herself to the hospital for treatment. The priority intervention is:
   a. Asking the patient if she wants to call the police.
   b. Providing information about a women's shelter.
   c. Providing information about domestic abuse services.
   d. Providing wound care to the injuries.

47. The psychiatric and mental health nurse has noted a number of nursing diagnoses in the plan of care for a patient with antisocial personality disorder admitted to the psychiatric unit under court order. The nursing diagnosis that should have priority is:
   a. Ineffective coping.
   b. Risk for other-directed violence.
   c. Low self-esteem.
   d. Impaired social interaction.

48. In the cycle of battering, during the phase of tension building, a battered woman typically:
   a. tries to hide.
   b. acts compliant.
   c. feels guilty.
   d. provokes abuse.

49. A patient who smoked two to three packs of cigarettes daily for over 20 years has been admitted to a no-smoking facility, so the psychiatric and mental health nurse is concerned about withdrawal symptoms. The most appropriate approach is:
   a. Providing smoking cessation classes.
   b. Allowing scheduled smoking.
   c. Providing emotional support.
   d. Providing nicotine patches.

50. When taking a history of a 65-year-old patient, the psychiatric and mental health nurse notes that the patient does not always seem to understand the questions, asks frequently for clarification, and speaks in an inappropriately loud tone of voice. Based on these observations, the psychiatric and mental health nurse recommends:
   a. cognitive assessment.
   b. alcohol screening.
   c. hearing assessment.
   d. drug screening.

51. A patient in treatment for substance abuse has a nursing diagnosis of *chronic low self-esteem.* An appropriate outcome criterion for this nursing diagnosis is:
    a. Patient exhibits no signs of substance intoxication or withdrawal.
    b. Patient can verbalize names of support people willing to help.
    c. Patient can verbalize positive self-characteristics.
    d. Patient can verbalize coping strategies to avoid substance abuse.

52. The psychiatric facility is using the recovery model for treatment, but one of the patients has indicated that she does not plan to continue taking lithium for her bipolar disorder. The most appropriate response for the psychiatric and mental health nurse is to:
    a. Insist that the patient continue taking the medication.
    b. Educate the patient about the need for medication.
    c. Warn the patient that she will suffer relapse without medication.
    d. Transition the patient to a different model for treatment.

53. A 15-year-old patient with autism spectrum disorder and obsessive-compulsive disorder rarely verbalizes except for occasional words that seem random, and the patient often becomes very agitated when the psychiatric and mental health nurse attempts to interact or communicate with him. The most appropriate method to improve communication is to:
    a. Keep interactions to a minimum to avoid agitating the patient.
    b. Have the patient evaluated by a speech therapist.
    c. Observe the patient carefully to note any communication strategies.
    d. Meet with parents/caregivers to discuss the patient's communication.

54. A patient with cognitive decline associated with dementia is undergoing sensory stimulation therapy, which is based on the concept of:
    a. neural plasticity.
    b. health promotion.
    c. behaviorism.
    d. recovery model.

55. A patient tells the psychiatric and mental health nurse that she is using aromatherapy to relieve anxiety and that she finds it more effective than medication. The most appropriate response is:
    a. "There's no evidence that aromatherapy works."
    b. "You should not stop taking the medication."
    c. "The aromatherapy may help you to relax."
    d. "If aromatherapy cures your anxiety, that's great!"

56. When utilizing psychodrama as a psychosocial therapy, the role of the *protagonist* is assumed by the:
    a. patient.
    b. nurse.
    c. therapist.
    d. family member.

57. A patient hospitalized with depression has a long history of alcoholism. Five days after admission, the patient exhibits increasing agitation, tremors, and confusion. The patient is disoriented and having hallucinations. Temperature, pulse, and blood pressure levels are elevated, and the patient is diaphoretic. The treatment that is most indicated is:
　　a. phenobarbital.
　　b. diazepam.
　　c. phenytoin.
　　d. clonidine.

58. Which of the following ethnic groups may require lower dosages of benzodiazepines and tricyclic antidepressants because of enzyme deficiencies that decrease the rate of metabolism?
　　a. Caucasians
　　b. Hispanics
　　c. African Americans
　　d. Asians

59. Which of the following drug types is most indicated for treatment of generalized anxiety disorder?
　　a. SSRI
　　b. Tricyclic antidepressant
　　c. Benzodiazepine
　　d. MAO inhibitor

60. When developing a plan of care for a patient with obsessive-compulsive disorder who compulsively washes his hands, the first goal in assisting the patient to reduce this ritualistic behavior and to increase coping skills is to assist the patient to:
　　a. Recognize precipitating factors.
　　b. Control the urge to carry out ritualistic behavior.
　　c. Analyze the underlying cause of the ritualistic behavior.
　　d. View the ritualistic behavior rationally.

61. As part of milieu therapy, the psychiatric and mental health nurse should expect to:
　　a. Provide weekly patient feedback.
　　b. Attend regular community meetings.
　　c. Direct patient participation.
　　d. Establish rules of patient behavior.

62. When using cognitive behavioral therapy for treatment of mood disorders, the focus is on:
　　a. rewarding positive behavior.
　　b. learning self-control.
　　c. making decisions about care.
　　d. changing automatic thoughts.

63. A patient who has not responded well to other antipsychotics is started on quetiapine. In the initial period when the patient's medication dosage is being adjusted, the patient should be assisted with:
　　a. ambulation.
　　b. toileting.
　　c. dressing.
　　d. eating.

64. A patient taking clozapine for treatment should be regularly monitored for:
    a. liver function.
    b. leukopenia.
    c. renal function.
    d. hypoglycemia.

65. Which of the following actions is most likely to be effective in establishing a relationship of trust with a newly admitted patient?
    a. Administering patient medications
    b. Providing the patient a list of unit rules
    c. Explaining the reason for unit procedures
    d. Giving the patient a tour of the facility

66. Which of the following is a boundary violation on the part of the psychiatric and mental health nurse?
    a. Accepting a box of candy to be shared by the staff
    b. Finding a patient attractive
    c. Holding the hand of a frightened patient
    d. Telling a patient about breaking up with a fiancé

67. A patient tends to walk and sit in a slumped over position, keeping the head and eyes down, and rarely making eye contact or initiating conversation. The patient responds with a low tone of voice. These behaviors most likely represent:
    a. dislike.
    b. low self-esteem.
    c. fear.
    d. anxiety.

68. During a meeting between a patient and the nurse, the patient paces back and forth and appears agitated and upset. Which of the following is the most appropriate response?
    a. "Why are you so upset?"
    b. "Take a moment and calm down before we proceed."
    c. "I notice you are pacing and seem upset."
    d. "Your pacing is making me uncomfortable."

69. A new patient on the unit has a speech impediment. During group therapy, some of the other participants made fun of her and mimicked her impediment, causing the patient to become very upset. Which of the following is an empathic response to the patient?
    a. "I know how you feel. I get so angry when people make fun of my ears."
    b. "You feel angry and sad about the other patients making fun of you."
    c. "Just ignore what the others say!'
    d. "The other patients made fun of you because they are insecure."

70. During which stage of the therapeutic relationship does the nurse examine personal feelings about working with a patient?
    a. Pre-interaction
    b. Orientation
    c. Working
    d. Termination

71. When a psychiatric and mental health nurse has difficulty setting limits on a patient's behavior because of an emotional response to a patient, this is an example of:
   a. transference.
   b. counter transference.
   c. magnification.
   d. codependency.

72. A patient is upset that he hasn't been able to complete a task successfully. Which of the following is an example of a *non-therapeutic* communication response?
   a. "I don't think you need to worry about that."
   b. "You're feeling frustrated."
   c. "Perhaps we can work on this together."
   d. "Let's talk about how you are feeling."

73. In group therapy, a patient called another patient "stupid and ugly," causing the second patient to begin crying. The psychiatric and mental health nurse meets with the first patient to discuss the behavior. The feedback that is most descriptive and focused on behavior is:
   a. "Mary was upset and sad when you called her 'stupid and ugly.'"
   b. "You were mean and rude when you called Mary 'stupid and ugly.'"
   c. "You should apologize for hurting Mary."
   d. "How would you feel if Mary had called you 'stupid and ugly'?"

74. A patient experienced a severe emotional crisis after her only child left home for college. This type of crisis is classified as:
   a. maturational/developmental.
   b. dispositional.
   c. traumatic stress.
   d. an anticipated life transition.

75. With the four-phase crisis intervention (Aguilera, 1998) method, which corresponds to the nursing process, which of the following actions should be completed during Phase 4 (evaluation/anticipatory planning)?
   a. Identify external support systems (family, friends, social agencies)
   b. Discuss how the patient will deal with triggering events in the future
   c. Assess the patient's personal perception of strengths
   d. Identify the precipitating event that caused the crisis

76. A patient is scheduled for electroconvulsive therapy for severe depression unresponsive to antidepressants. The pre-procedure medication that the nurse anticipates giving is a(n):
   a. sedative.
   b. analgesic.
   c. cholinergic blocking agent.
   d. muscle relaxant.

77. A patient with intermittent explosive disorder is exhibiting the prodromal syndrome of escalation of anger. The most appropriate first step in preventing an act of violence is to:
    a. Ensure adequate staff are available.
    b. Utilize seclusion or restraints.
    c. Attempt to talk the patient down.
    d. Offer medication to the patient.

78. A patient has undergone electroconvulsive therapy (ECT) and is awakening from the anesthesia. The initial patient response that is most expected is:
    a. sedation.
    b. memory impairment.
    c. agitation.
    d. anger.

79. A patient flirts with her male nurse and then complains to the administrative staff that the nurse is "coming on" to her. This is an example of:
    a. sublimation.
    b. suppression.
    c. displacement.
    d. projection.

80. A male patient who acts very polite and considerate in the presence of other patients and staff makes threatening and vulgar sexual comments to the psychiatric and mental health nurse when no one else can hear. The most appropriate method of reporting this behavior is to:
    a. File an incident report.
    b. Document exactly what the patient said and the circumstances in the nursing notes.
    c. Document that the patient was "behaving inappropriately" in the nursing notes.
    d. Report the situation to the administrator.

81. A patient became very angry with the group leader in a therapy session and threw a glass of water at the leader. Which of the following statements by the patient suggests that the patient is using the ego defense mechanism of *rationalization* to explain the actions?
    a. "I didn't throw the glass. It slipped out of my hand."
    b. "I lost my temper and threw the glass!"
    c. "The leader repeatedly egged me on, forcing me to act."
    d. "I'm very sorry about throwing the glass of water."

82. The purpose of the Substance Abuse and Mental Health Services Administration's (SAMHSA's) *Opening Doors* program is to:
    a. Prevent and end homelessness.
    b. Promote mental health care for veterans.
    c. Provide residential care for the mentally ill.
    d. Prevent prescription drug misuse and abuse.

83. A patient with PTSD is employed but has not disclosed his condition to his employer. He feels overwhelmed by the work schedule and wants accommodations, but when he requested a more flexible schedule, he was denied. His most appropriate course of action is to:
    a. Get a different job.
    b. File a suit against the employer.
    c. Seek further treatment to reduce anxiety.
    d. Disclose that he has a disability.

84. A patient who suffered severe brain damage as a result of a suicide attempt had written an advance directive stating that "no heroic measures" be used to keep her alive; however, the patient is being maintained on life support at the family's insistence. As an advocate for the patient, the most appropriate response for the psychiatric and mental health nurse is to:
    a. File a complaint with the district attorney.
    b. Remain supportive and provide education to family.
    c. Tell the physician that he is violating the patient's rights.
    d. File a complaint with the hospital administration.

85. Which of the following gives patients the right to access their medical records and to have corrections made?
    a. OSHA
    b. ADA
    c. HIPAA
    d. NAMI

86. According to the International Society of Psychiatric-Mental Health Nurses (ISPN) position paper "Emergency Care Psychiatric Clinical Framework," clinical assessment of the patient in the emergency department should begin with:
    a. a focused medical assessment.
    b. a mental status exam.
    c. a review of current medications.
    d. safety concerns.

87. The nursing organization that is the most active politically, lobbying to promote the interests of the nursing profession and policies regarding health care reform, is the:
    a. American Nurses Credentialing Center (ANCC).
    b. American Nurses Association (ANA).
    c. American Psychiatric Nurses Association (APNA).
    d. American Association of Colleges of Nursing (AACN).

88. The most effective position for active listening is:
    a. Sitting beside the patient, touching the patient's arm.
    b. Standing near the patient with arms uncrossed.
    c. Sitting directly in front of the patient with arms uncrossed.
    d. Position is irrelevant.

89. A caregiver states that she is exhausted and angry about the quality of her life because of having to constantly care for her mother, who has severe Alzheimer's disease. The most appropriate initial recommendation is:

    a. family/friend assistance.
    b. a long-term care facility.
    c. a support group.
    d. respite care.

90. The legislative act that provides access to community services for older adults and Native Americans, including meals, legal assistance, adult day care, and transportation, is the:

    a. Older Americans Act (OAA).
    b. Americans with Disabilities Act (ADA).
    c. Omnibus Budget Reconciliation Act (OBRA).
    d. Affordable Care Act (ACA).

91. When a patient thinks, "If I stop drinking, I can repair my marriage," this type of "self-talk" is referred to as:

    a. uncertainty maintenance.
    b. uncertainty reduction.
    c. realistic goal setting.
    d. learner readiness.

92. When using Keller's (1987) attention-relevance-confidence-satisfaction (ARCS) model as a motivational strategy for learners, which term refers to the use of variable instructional methods?

    a. Attention
    b. Relevance
    c. Confidence
    d. Satisfaction

93. When assessing the learning needs of a patient to promote self-care, the need that should have priority is:

    a. pain control.
    b. anxiety reduction.
    c. dietary instruction.
    d. disease pathology.

94. When teaching, the psychiatric and mental health nurse tries to relate new information to knowledge that patients already have in memory to improve memory retention. This type of encoding is:

    a. visual.
    b. organizational.
    c. spontaneous/automatic.
    d. elaborative.

95. The patient's coping mechanism is a factor in which type of readiness to learn?

    a. Emotional
    b. Physical
    c. Experiential
    d. Knowledge

96. The psychiatric and mental health nurse is providing education about coping mechanisms to a group of patients, one of whom has recently developed profound hearing loss but is unable to utilize sign language. Much of the prepared material is in video format. The most appropriate accommodation for the patient with hearing loss is:
    a. Provide closed-captioning for the videos.
    b. Print out a script of the video.
    c. Provide illustrations and written explanations.
    d. Separate this patient from the group and instruct privately.

97. When the psychiatric and mental health nurse is serving as a preceptor for a student, the primary responsibility is:
    a. Providing supervision to the student.
    b. Preventing errors in nursing care.
    c. Evaluating and assigning grades.
    d. Teaching and promoting learning.

98. Which of the following is the key ingredient in developing a learning contract with a patient?
    a. Cognitive ability
    b. Trust
    c. Motivation
    d. Developmental stage

99. The psychiatric and mental health nurse should recommend that adults with a history of illicit injection drug use get the following vaccination(s):
    a. Hepatitis A and Hepatitis B
    b. Pneumococcal polysaccharide (PPSV23)
    c. Meningococcal
    d. Human papillomavirus

100. When serving as a mentor to a newly hired nurse, the psychiatric and mental health nurse noted that the new nurse became intimidated by an aggressive patient and was ineffectual in dealing with the patient's behavior. The psychiatric and mental health nurse's most appropriate response to the nurse is:
    a. "You didn't handle that situation with the patient very well."
    b. "What do you think you did wrong in that situation?"
    c. "Always call for help if you don't know what to do with a patient."
    d. "How do you think you might have handled that differently?"

101. A patient being treated for depression has started an exercise program to help alleviate symptoms and plans to do muscle-building exercises at a gym twice weekly and to walk daily. How many total minutes of walking per week is the minimum recommendation?
    a. 60
    b. 100
    c. 150
    d. 200

102. According to the ANA, which of the following is a core principle of peer review?
    a. Peer review should be done anonymously.
    b. Peer review expectations are the same regardless of the nurse's developmental stage.
    c. Peer review should be done by a nurse's immediate supervisor.
    d. Peer review should focus on nursing practice.

103. The American Psychiatric Nurses Association (APNA) position statement on the use of seclusion and restraint states that:
    a. Seclusion and restraint should be routinely used to control aggressive behavior.
    b. Efforts should be made to reduce or eliminate the use of seclusion and restraint.
    c. Seclusion and restraint is generally under-utilized in psychiatric care.
    d. Restraints should be applied to minimize patient movement.

104. A patient deals with traumatic stress by accepting the stressful event, exposing herself to the stress by thinking about and describing the event, and working to understand the meaning of the event. This patient is engaged in:
    a. repressive coping.
    b. reframing.
    c. rational coping.
    d. stress inoculation training.

105. The psychiatric and mental health nurse has accepted a position in an area with a large Native American population. The psychiatric and mental health nurse expects that Native Americans are:
    a. Comfortable being touched by healthcare providers.
    b. Comfortable with small personal space.
    c. Comfortable with direct eye contact.
    d. Comfortable with silence during conversation.

106. On the psychiatric unit, patients are rewarded for desired behaviors by receiving tokens that can be exchanged for privileges. This is a technique that is used in:
    a. behavioral therapy.
    b. psychoanalytic therapy.
    c. cognitive therapy.
    d. Gestalt therapy.

107. A patient has a severe phobia about heights and is unwilling to fly in an airplane or to ascend beyond the ground floor of a building. The most effective treatment approach is likely:
    a. cognitive restructuring.
    b. mindfulness meditation.
    c. exposure therapy.
    d. a self-help group.

108. A patient who is fearful about interacting with others attempts to change her perception by imagining that the others are afraid to interact with her. The strategy that the patient is utilizing is:
    a. assertiveness.
    b. reframing.
    c. repressive coping.
    d. intellectualism.

109. A patient with antisocial personality disorder has very poor social skills and resents authority. Which of the following therapeutic approaches may be most effective?
    a. Cognitive behavioral therapy
    b. Psychoanalytic therapy
    c. Psychopharmacology
    d. Milieu therapy

110. Which of the following National Alliance on Mental Illness (NAMI) programs is especially designed to provide strategies for caregiving for parents/caregivers of children or adolescents with mental illness?
    a. Peer-to-Peer
    b. Homefront
    c. Basics
    d. Family-to-Family

111. Under the American Nurses Association (ANA) *Code of Ethics*, if the psychiatric and mental health nurse feels that a research project is morally objectionable, the nurse has the right to:
    a. Lodge a criminal complaint.
    b. Refuse to participate.
    c. Stop the research project.
    d. Ask the ANA to evaluate the project.

112. When conducting a community assessment for preventive measures as part of community-based care, the three primary factors to consider are:
    a. People, environment, and social systems.
    b. People, costs, and time.
    c. Time, environment, and costs.
    d. Social systems, needs, and costs.

113. A patient who has been homeless is to be discharged. When developing a discharge plan with the patient, the psychiatric and mental health nurse should:
    a. Provide a list of local shelters to the patient.
    b. Contact local shelters to secure a place for the patient.
    c. Ask the patient where he plans to stay after discharge.
    d. Tell the patient to contact shelters before discharge.

114. A 30-year-old patient with a 6-year-old child is treated in an outpatient clinic. The patient often has little money for food and purchases inexpensive non-nutritious fast food. The most appropriate recommendation is:
    a. home delivery of meals (Meals-on-Wheels).
    b. nutritional counseling.
    c. WIC.
    d. local food banks.

115. A patient who is morbidly obese (>400 pounds) has frequently binged on food, eating until she vomits. Which community resource or support group is likely to be most helpful?
    a. Weight Watchers®
    b. Home meal delivery (Meals-on-Wheels)
    c. Overeaters Anonymous®
    d. Recovery International®

116. When interacting with a patient who is vision-impaired, the psychiatric and mental health nurse should:
    a. Introduce others who are present by giving their names and roles.
    b. Explain and describe actions as they are being carried out.
    c. Hold the patient's hand when addressing the patient.
    d. Always stand in front of the patient when addressing the patient.

117. A patient who is being admitted to an outpatient program for recovering cocaine abusers states that he has a history of gonorrhea and chlamydia, has multiple sex partners, and uses condoms erratically, especially if he has been drinking. The most appropriate initial screening for the patient is for:
    a. sexual addiction.
    b. hepatitis.
    c. sexually-transmitted diseases.
    d. alcohol abuse.

118. A patient's plan of care calls for the patient to attend an outpatient therapy group for preventing drug abuse relapse, but the patient's insurance will not reimburse the costs of participation. Which of the following is likely the most appropriate alternative when modifying the plan of care?
    a. Refer the patient to Narcotics Anonymous®
    b. Provide literature about preventive measures
    c. Refer the patient to online resources
    d. Provide the patient with staff contact information

119. A female patient with a methadone overdose is undergoing Q-T monitoring. The normal range for the Q-T interval is:
    a. 0.33 to 0.35 seconds.
    b. 0.36 to 0.44 seconds.
    c. 0.45 to 0.50 seconds.
    d. 0.51 to 0.53 seconds.

120. When videotaping patients in a secure unit for safety reasons, which areas may be videotaped without patient permission in most states?
    a. Any areas within the unit
    b. Patients' bedrooms only
    c. All areas except for the patient's bathroom
    d. Public areas within the unit

121. A patient becomes confused during the night and falls when getting out of bed. The most appropriate solution to prevent further falls is:
    a. Apply a pressure-sensitive movement pad with an alarm.
    b. Place physical restraints on the patient.
    c. Provide a sitter in the room with the patient.
    d. Move the patient's bed to a room next to the nursing desk.

122. A patient with severe treatment-resistant depression has had a device implanted in the chest wall for vagus nerve stimulation (VNS). When educating the patient about the treatment, the psychiatric and mental health nurse tells the patient to expect improvement in symptoms:
    a. almost immediately.
    b. within a few days.
    c. within a few weeks.
    d. within a few months.

123. Which of the following would fit the National Quality Forum's definition of a "serious reportable event?"
    a. Patient commits suicide two weeks after discharge from the hospital.
    b. Patient elopes from the hospital and is killed when running into traffic.
    c. Patient attempts suicide in the hospital but has only minor injuries.
    d. Patient falls in the hospital, resulting in a small abrasion on the hip.

124. Data show that patients discharged during the day shift, 8 am to 4 pm, have better compliance with follow-up than patients discharged after 4 pm, suggesting a quality variance in discharge procedures. Which of the following is most likely to result in variance reduction?
    a. Notifying the afternoon staff that discharge procedures are deficient.
    b. Rewarding the day staff for quality discharge procedures.
    c. Providing a discharge checklist that is to be utilized with all patients.
    d. Rewarding all staff for meeting goals of variance reduction.

125. A patient taking an SSRI has become quite agitated and exhibits myoclonus, hyperreflexia, coarse tremors, diaphoresis, tachycardia, confusion, dilated pupils, fever, and diarrhea. Based on these symptoms, the psychiatric and mental health nurses suspects:
    a. delirium.
    b. meningitis.
    c. serotonin syndrome.
    d. tardive dyskinesia.

126. A patient who had been treated as an inpatient for bulimia nervosa has been discharged and states on follow-up that she has not had any distorted eating or purging. Which of the following findings suggests that the patient has resumed purging?
    a. Potassium: 3.2 mEq/L
    b. Potassium: 3.7 mEq/L
    c. Serum amylase: 45 U/L
    d. Chloride: 102 mEq/L

127. A patient who had a spontaneous abortion resulting from drug abuse becomes very upset when talking about it with the psychiatric and mental health nurse and begins to cry. The most appropriate response is to:
    a. Tell the patient she is obviously upset that she caused the abortion.
    b. Suggest the patient focus on the future and changing her behavior.
    c. Hug the patient to provide comfort while she is crying.
    d. Sit quietly with the patient, allowing her to express feelings.

128. Which of the following is an appropriate task for the psychiatric and mental health nurse to delegate to unlicensed assistive personnel (UAP)?
    a. Take vital signs for the initial admission physical examination.
    b. Apply physical restraints to a patient as per physician's orders.
    c. Monitor a patient's intake of food during a meal.
    d. Administer a laxative to a patient.

129. Which of the following is the best approach when obtaining a history of an adolescent?
    a. Conduct the interview without the parents/caregivers present.
    b. Ask the adolescent if the parents/caregivers should remain during the interview.
    c. Ask the parents/caregivers if they want to be present for the interview.
    d. Conduct the interview with the parents/caregivers present.

130. Which of the following statements or questions by a psychiatric and mental health nurse about a patient who identifies as transgender (male to female) suggests the nurse's attitude may negatively impact delivery of care to the patient?
    a. "I don't really understand what transgender means."
    b. "I believe that someone born a man is always a man."
    c. "Should I refer to the patient as he or she?"
    d. "I try to treat everyone the same."

131. A patient becomes extremely agitated during an activity and begins yelling and banging his head against the wall. The first step in de-escalation is to:
    a. Remove other patients from the environment.
    b. Have a team of staff members exhibit a show of force.
    c. Utilize a third-person "negotiator" to calm the patient.
    d. Call for physical restraints to be applied.

132. A 15-year-old patient with anorexia nervosa has responded well to therapy and has gained about 2 pounds per week. As part of the plan of care, the patient will begin to participate in an eating disorder support group. One of the disadvantages of the patient's attending a support group is:
    a. Most patients in support groups are older.
    b. The patient may be too immature to benefit from a support group.
    c. The patient no longer needs support because of weight gain.
    d. The patient may be exposed to other patients with more severe symptoms.

133. When utilizing Focus Charting® for documentation of the nursing process, the focus may be on:
    a. medical diagnosis.
    b. routine daily therapy.
    c. current patient behavior.
    d. the patient's history.

134. A suicidal patient refuses to stay beyond the 72-hour hold in the inpatient unit because of lack of insurance and is to be followed on an outpatient basis. When developing the interdisciplinary plan for discharge, the most important consideration is:
    a. the patient will sign a no-suicide contract.
    b. the patient will not be left alone.
    c. the family will check the patient's apartment to remove dangerous items.
    d. follow-up appointments will be scheduled.

135. A patient with psychotic behavior is transferred from a board and care facility to the psychiatric unit for treatment. The transfer form has nothing listed under "current medications." Based on this finding, the psychiatric and mental health nurse should:
    a. Ask the patient if he has been taking medications.
    b. Assume the patient has been taking no medications.
    c. Ask the psychiatrist if the patient has been taking medications.
    d. Contact the board and care facility to verify the information.

136. A 68-year-old Medicare patient who is to be discharged from a mental health facility wants to be followed by home health care rather than to return to the clinic for outpatient treatment. Which of the following may make the patient eligible for home health care?
    a. The patient has a debilitating physical condition that makes travel difficult.
    b. The patient doesn't want to waste time traveling to and from the clinic.
    c. The patient does not have a car and must depend on public transportation.
    d. The patient is over 65 years old.

137. The three primary components of panic control treatment (PCT) include:
    a. Imagery, progressive relaxation exercises, and cognitive restructuring.
    b. Cognitive restructuring, in vivo exposure, and interoceptive exposure.
    c. Assessment, in vivo exposure, and evaluation.
    d. Progressive relaxation, cognitive restructuring, and in vivo exposure.

138. Which of the following tools is frequently utilized for drug evaluation at the beginning of treatment with anti-anxiety drugs, as well as during treatment to adjust dosage and determine outcomes?
    a. Hamilton Anxiety Rating Scale
    b. Psychological Screening Inventory
    c. Milton Clinical Multiaxial Inventory
    d. Beck Anxiety Inventory.

139. Which characteristic is typical of a patient presenting with a suspected conversion disorder, such as a sudden sensory or motor deficit?
    a. Patient exhibits lack of concern about the impairment
    b. Patient exhibits very typical symptoms and pathology
    c. The more the patient knows, the more bizarre the symptoms
    d. Patient is typically very well educated and knowledgeable

140. A patient is undergoing habit reversal therapy (HRT) as part of the interdisciplinary plan of care for trichotillomania. Which of the following actions by the patient indicates the patient is carrying out the *competitive response* step to control urges?
   a. The patient identifies and creates a list of triggers
   b. The patient keeps a detailed list of all urge behaviors
   c. The patient states she knows she doesn't need to give in to urges
   d. The patient taps her wrist with an index finger when she has an urge

141. A patient with severe anxiety has persistent negative thoughts, believing that others think she is ugly and stupid. The patient's interdisciplinary plan of care calls for use of Acceptance Commitment Therapy (ACT). Which of the following actions by the patient indicates that the patient is successfully carrying out *cognitive defusion* during an anxiety attack?
   a. The patient uses distraction to stop thinking negative thoughts
   b. The patient uses imagery to relax and to control negative thoughts
   c. The patient states that she understands she shouldn't react to thoughts
   d. The patient makes a list of evidence regarding the truth of negative thoughts

142. A patient who is undergoing Motivational Enhancement Therapy (MET) for treatment of substance abuse has made a decision to change behavior and stop using, indicating the patient is at the stage of:
   a. pre-contemplation.
   b. contemplation.
   c. determination.
   d. action.

143. A patient who uses problem-solving skills and coping strategies to deal with stressful situations, such as illness, is exhibiting:
   a. resilience.
   b. resourcefulness.
   c. self-efficacy.
   d. hardiness.

144. A patient with depression has been very withdrawn and is avoiding any socialization with others, but the psychiatric and mental health nurse notes that the patient sat with two other patients during a concert, occasionally speaking to them. The most appropriate feedback to the patient is:
   a. "I noticed you were sitting with other patients during the concert."
   b. "I was so happy to see you interacting with other patients at the concert!"
   c. "Why did you decide to sit with other patients?"
   d. "Sitting with the other patients is a good sign that you are improving."

145. Which physiological response is common when patients are undergoing acute withdrawal from opioids?
   a. Hypertension
   b. Hypotension
   c. Somnolence
   d. Constipation

146. A patient has been started on disulfiram before discharge from a treatment facility for alcoholism. A friend comes to visit the patient, and within about 5 minutes of the friend's leaving, the patient becomes hypotensive, complains of severe chest pain, headache, and vertigo, and begins vomiting copiously. The most likely reason is:
    a. an adverse reaction to disulfiram.
    b. acetaldehyde syndrome.
    c. delirium tremens.
    d. serotonin syndrome.

147. When educating a patient who has been prescribed an MAO inhibitor, the psychiatric and mental health nurse advises the patient to avoid:
    a. oranges.
    b. low-fat milk.
    c. chicken (white meat).
    d. aged cheese (such as Swiss).

148. The psychiatric and mental health nurse is assigning nursing diagnoses to a patient with obsessive-compulsive disorder. Which nursing diagnosis is appropriate to account for the patient's ritualistic behavior and obsessive thoughts?
    a. Ineffective role performance
    b. Social isolation
    c. Ineffective coping
    d. Powerlessness

149. Following a hurricane that leveled a woman's home, the woman goes to an emergency shelter and exhibits severe anxiety when interviewed by the psychiatric and mental health nurse, who is part of the emergency response team. The most appropriate intervention is:
    a. Provide anti-anxiety medication to reduce the woman's symptoms.
    b. Provide reassurance and discussion of the stages of grief.
    c. Ask family or friends to stay with the woman.
    d. Tell the woman that she is safe and everything will be all right.

150. One of the most important goals of family-focused psychoeducational (FFP) treatment for bipolar disorder is for family members to learn to:
    a. use positive reinforcement.
    b. manage the patient's medications.
    c. set behavioral limits.
    d. recognize early warning signs of relapse.

Answers and Explanations

1. **B:** Patients who have been raped are often severely traumatized emotionally as well as physically and are commonly very fearful and panicked, so the first thing that the mental health nurse should communicate is "You are safe here. No one can hurt you." The psychiatric and mental health nurse may need to repeat this a number of times because traumatized patients may block out what people are saying. The nurse should also reassure the patient that the attack was not the patient's fault and that the nurse is sorry for what the patient has gone through.

2. **D:** Because the patient is intimidated by her spouse and has stated she is afraid to stand up to him, as an advocate for the patient, the nurse should notify the physician of the patient's feelings about the treatment. Being coerced into signing a consent form is not the same as giving informed consent, which is required by law. Because patients are vulnerable to manipulation, the nurse must ensure that the actual wishes of the patient are respected.

3. **C:** The most likely reason the patient was able to read slowly but not state what she had read is low health literacy. The ability to read is different from the ability to comprehend, and comprehension usually lags behind reading skills by about three grade levels. Thus, a person who is able to read at the fourth-grade level may have only a first-grade reading comprehension, making it difficult for the person to understand health materials, especially since the vocabulary is often more difficult to understand than that found in other readings.

4. **A:** The patient is using the ego defense mechanism of **denial** when the patient, who has had repeated arrests for driving under the influence of alcohol, refuses to admit that he has a drinking problem and states that the police have targeted him unfairly. **Reaction formation** is refusing to acknowledge undesirable feelings, thoughts, or behavior by exaggerating the opposite. **Regression** is retreating to an earlier level of development. **Undoing** is carrying out an action to negate a previous unacceptable one.

5. **B:** The patient's delusions are interfering with development at the level of love/belonging needs. Maslow's hierarchy of needs is based on the premise that one must satisfy one type of need before one can attain the next. The hierarchy of needs includes:
   - Physiological: Basic needs such as air, food, water, shelter.
   - Safety and Security: Freedom from fear; physical comfort, safety.
   - Love and belonging: Companionship, giving/receiving love, group identification, satisfying interpersonal relationships.
   - Self-esteem: Working for success, desiring respect and prestige, seeking self-respect.
   - Self-actualization: Feeling of self-fulfillment, satisfaction with achievements.

6. **D:** Kava is contraindicated because of safety issues and can result in liver damage, so the patient should have liver function tests completed. Early signs of liver damage include fatigue and dark urine. Some people may exhibit jaundice as well. Amitriptyline is broken down by the liver, so kava may increase the rate at which that occurs, also increasing the adverse effects of the drug. Kava, which has been used in the past for anxiety, may increase depression.

7. **C:** Erikson postulated that the stage of adulthood, generativity versus stagnation, is characterized by achieving the personal life goals that the person had formulated. The eight development stages include:
   - Trust vs. mistrust (Infancy, 0 to 18 months).

- Autonomy vs. shame and doubt (Early childhood, 18 months to 3 years).
- Initiative vs. guilt (Late childhood, 3-6 years).
- Industry vs. inferiority (School age, 6-12 years).
- Identity vs. role confusion (Adolescence, 12-20 years).
- Intimacy vs. isolation (Young adulthood, 20-30 years).
- Generativity vs. stagnation (Adulthood, 30-65 years).
- Ego integrity vs. despair (65 years-death).

8. B: Four different mental health associations came together to create the International Society of Psychiatric-Mental Health Nurses in 1999. These four associations became divisions of the new organization:
- Association of Child and Adolescent Psychiatric Nurses (ACAPN)
- International Society of Psychiatric Consultation Liaison Nurses (ISPCLN)
- Society of Education and Research in Psychiatric Mental Health Nursing (SERPN)
- Adult and Geropsychiatric Mental Health Nurses (AGPN)

The purpose of the ISPN includes promoting quality care, outlining essential educational requirements, promoting research, and developing health care policy.

9. D: AHRQ's *You Can Quit Smoking* guide includes five steps:
1. Getting ready: Considering past attempts (successes/failures) and setting a date for quitting cold turkey.
2. Getting support/encouragement: Telling others and contacting support groups/helplines.
3. Learning new skills/behaviors: Drinking plenty of water, establishing new habits, practicing distractions, and reducing stress.
4. Getting and using medication correctly: Obtaining nicotine replacement or other medications as needed.
5. Preparing for relapse/difficult situations: Avoiding other smokers and alcohol or situations that trigger desire for cigarettes. Eating well and living a healthy lifestyle.

10. C: A score of 18 out of 30 on the MMSS usually indicates moderate cognitive impairment. Scores of 27 to 30 indicate normal cognition while 10 to 18 indicate moderate cognitive impairment. Scores may be affected by numerous variables (age, hearing, intelligence, vision, physical condition), so the MMSE score alone is not adequate for diagnosis of dementia. However, it is a good guide, and those with very low scores (≤9) usually demonstrate severe cognitive impairment.

11. D: A patient who is severely depressed may not give complete answers or may even be reluctant to talk, but the psychiatric and mental health nurse should progress with the history and physical exam in a supportive manner. If the patient does not respond to open-ended questions, such as "How can we help you?" then the psychiatric and mental health nurse may need to use close-ended questions, such as "Have you attempted suicide?" which require short responses. The psychiatric and mental health nurse should remain non-judgmental in affect and tone of voice, understanding that some information regarding history may need to be obtained at a later time.

12. A: Piaget's theory of cognitive development in children applies to adults in relation to readiness to learn. Like the child, the adult can incorporate new learning experiences through assimilation and goes through changes in dealing with these experiences through accommodation. Piaget stressed the idea that a child must be developmentally ready for learning and that trying to teach a child who is not ready may result in rote memorization but not real learning. These same concepts can apply equally to adult learning.

13. B: The brief mental status evaluation typically includes questions to evaluate the patient's orientation to time and place, recent memory, and the ability to comprehend spatial relationships and to use language. Other mental functions include:

- Ability to concentrate: Ask the patient to spell the word "world" in reverse.
- Ability to follow verbal commands: Ask the patient to carry out a two- to three-step task.
- Ability to utilize abstract thinking: Ask the patient what "A stitch in time saves nine" means.
- Attention/immediate recall: List three objects and ask the patient to repeat the list immediately and again in a few minutes.

14. A: Developmental milestones that usually occur during adolescence (12 to 18 years) include:

- Understanding abstract concepts.
- Achieving adult stature and sexual maturity: Growth spurt for females peaks at about age 11.5 and for boys at about age 13.5. The average age of menarche is 12 and onset of nocturnal emissions is 13.5.
- Developing secondary sexual characteristics.
- Desiring acceptance from peers.
- Expressing concern about body image.
- Developing romantic attractions to the opposite or same gender.
- Showing increasing desire for independence from parents.

15. C: Mindfulness meditation is a technique used in cognitive therapy, which focuses on assisting the patient to correct distorted thinking and to consider the meaning of events rather than focusing on behavior. Techniques include cognitive restructuring in which patients are advised to consider evidence for and against specific beliefs in order to deal more effectively with outcomes. Mindfulness meditation teaches the patient to be aware of feelings and emotions "in the moment" in order to detect symptoms before they become problematic.

16. D: Forgetting to keep an appointment is an example of normal cognitive changes associated with aging. Patients may remember events or stories but forget details about them or may misplace items, such as keys or jewelry; however, if people completely forget events, such as attending a party, forget important things, such as where savings accounts are located, or forget how to do something that the person has done previously for long periods of time, such as using the stove to cook, then this is often an indication of dementia.

17. B: The HEEADSSS method:

- H—Home environment: Where patient lives and with whom, as well as living situation.
- E—Education/employment: Description of school, bullying, grades, work schedule/place.
- E—Eating: Concerns about body appearance, weight, recent weight changes, dieting.
- A—Activities (peer-related): Free time, online, sports, clubs, friends.
- D—Drugs: Use of alcohol, tobacco, or drugs by patient or friends.
- S—Sexuality: Romantic relationships, sexual activity, contraceptives, pregnancy.
- S—Suicide/Depression: Stress, sadness, boredom, insomnia, bullying, suicidal ideation, suicide attempts.
- S—Safety: Injuries, seat belt use, texting while driving, meeting strangers online, riding with impaired driver, violence in school/area.

18. C: When using the reflective method during an interview, the psychiatric and mental health nurse reflects back or repeats what the patient has just said. In this case, if the patient said that his

pain "moves around," the reflective response would be "moves around?" This encourages the patient to elaborate without the need for more direct questioning. The psychiatric and mental health nurse may also use facilitation—leaning forward, nodding the head, making eye contact, and saying "yes"—to encourage the patient to share information.

19. A: When reconciling a patient's medications, the psychiatric and mental health nurse should utilize all available information and begin by comparing different lists and then going over them in detail with the patient. Lists prepared by the physician may not include medications ordered by other physicians as patients often forget to provide this information to other healthcare providers. The psychiatric and mental health nurse should not depend on the lists alone but should prompt the patient for more information, as the patient may forget about some medications or think over-the-counter drugs and vitamins/herbs don't count.

20. C: When a patient reports chest pain, the psychiatric and mental health nurse should always probe for more information and ask the patient to show where the pain is. Typically, if pain is severe and crushing, as may occur with angina, the patient will indicate the site of the pain with the full hand or a fist, but running the finger up and down the sternal area suggests heartburn. Pleurisy is not usually felt in the sternal area, and gastritis may cause pain in the epigastrium.

21. D: Lithium has a narrow therapeutic range (0.6 to 1.4 mEq/L for adults), so this patient is exhibiting signs of mild lithium toxicity, which occurs with levels between 1.5 and 2.5 mEq/L. Patients may also exhibit muscle tremors and/or twitching, ataxia, tinnitus, blurred vision, and vertigo. Deep tendon reflexes may be hyperactive. Severe symptoms occur with levels above 2.5 mEq/L, characterized by elevated temperature, decreased urinary output (renal failure), hypotension, cardiac dysrhythmias, altered consciousness, coma, or death.

22. B: When planning a group discussion with patients, an important consideration when forming the group is that the group members have similar health literacy and conditions (or degrees of anxiety) because the leader must ensure that all members of the group have correctly interpreted and understood information being shared; this can be difficult if patients have a wide range of health literacy, anxiety, or conditions. However, some diversity is valuable because it allows for different perceptions and observations.

23. B: The patient is exhibiting possible signs of hypothyroidism—weight gain, lethargy, and feeling "chilled" or having increased sensitivity to cold—and should have thyroid function tests. Patients may also complain of poor concentration, constipation, dry hair, and somnolence and may exhibit bradycardia and joint or muscle pain. Hypothyroidism is a common cause of depression; it is often one of the first signs, and is typically overlooked. Hyperthyroidism may result in anxiety and emotional lability with some patients developing acute episodes of mania.

24. D: The psychiatric and mental health nurse should suspect that the patient has a urinary tract infection. In older adults, one of the first signs of a urinary tract infection may be sudden onset of confusion, as other usual signs (urinary frequency, burning) may be absent. The cause of the confusion is not clear but may relate to a combination of mild dehydration and fever. The patient should have a urinalysis and urine culture. The confusion usually clears rapidly with treatment for the infection.

25. C: A plan for relapse prevention must contain concrete actions: "I will call my sponsor if I feel like using again." The plan should focus on what the patient will do, not the family: "My family will make sure I don't relapse." The focus on family takes the responsibility away from the patient.

Statements indicating that the patient recognizes the need for a plan, such as "Don't worry, I've learned my lesson," and "I know I have to stop taking drugs," are not a plan.

26. B: Schizophrenia is characterized by both positive and negative symptoms. For a diagnosis of schizophrenia, the patient must exhibit at least one of three positive symptoms:
- Positive: Disorganized speech, hallucinations, and delusions.
- Negative: Flat affect, poor eye contact, impaired hygiene, social isolation, alogia (poverty of speech), apathy, and anhedonia (inability to experience pleasure).

Schizophrenia spectrum disorders now encompass what were previously considered different subtypes (such as paranoid schizophrenia). Two criteria A symptoms are required for a diagnosis of schizophrenia along with the positive symptom(s).

27. C: **Delusions of reference:** Patient believes that almost everything refers to himself, often believing that other people are constantly talking about him or laughing at him and that newspapers and TV programs are sending coded messages to him. **Delusions of grandeur:** Patient believes she has exceptional power or knowledge, such as believing she is Queen Elizabeth. **Delusions of persecution:** Patient believes others intend to harm him, such as believing he is being videotaped or recorded. **Delusions of control:** Patient believes others are controlling her, such as believing the doctor implanted something to control her mind.

28. A: Imagery and self-relaxation techniques are likely to be the most effective in providing relief from anxiety because these techniques can be learned easily and utilized whenever the patient feels stressed. Massage also has benefits in reducing anxiety but is expensive and not readily available during times of stress. Some people feel that aromatherapy (orange, bergamot, lavender) is beneficial. Studies regarding the use of acupuncture to relieve anxiety have been inconclusive, although some people feel it helps reduce anxiety.

29. B: **Clang associations:** Patient chooses words according to sound, often rhyming words, such as "The food is hot. I am hot and shot. The pot has been bought." **Word salad:** The patient strings together words randomly, such as "Many dogs green circle willingly." **Neologisms:** The patient creates new words that have meaning to the person but not to others, such as "I saw the magaraly." **Associative looseness:** The patient shifts topics from one to another with no connection between them, such as "I ate lunch, but the water was too dirty for swimming. Swimming is the way to the office."

30. D: Ego defense mechanisms:
- **Compensation:** Compensating for what the person perceives as a weakness (such as short stature) by emphasizing other traits or characteristics (martial arts, aggressive behavior).
- **Identification:** Taking on characteristics/behavior of someone the person admires or looks up to in order to increase feelings of self-worth.
- **Repression:** Blocking perceptions, memories, and feelings from conscious awareness.
- **Introjection:** Integrating belief systems/values of someone else into the person's own, the way children assume the value system of the parents.

31. C: The most appropriate response is the one that expresses acceptance of the person's belief along with reasonable doubt: "I understand you believe your room is bugged, but I don't believe it's possible." It's important to avoid denying outright that delusions are real ("That's not true....") or arguing with the patient ("Remember what you learned....") as this is not likely to change the

person's beliefs and will likely interfere with the therapeutic relationship. However, it's also important to avoid supporting the delusion ("Ok, let see if we can find the bug...").

32. A: The most appropriate response to a patient stating that she wants to die and has nothing to live for is "Do you have a suicide plan?" The psychiatric and mental health nurse should confront the issue directly in a matter-of-fact manner because this helps to convey to the patient that the nurse is willing to hear a truthful response, and when confronted in this way, patients are more likely to share plans. Patients who have actually developed a suicide plan are at increased risk.

33. D: The patient is exhibiting behavior and thought processes associated with social isolation by withdrawing from others, staying in his room, being preoccupied with his own thoughts, and feeling rejected. The outcome goal should be for the patient to voluntarily spend time with staff and other patients. The psychiatric and mental health nurse should make frequent brief contacts and provide positive reinforcement, showing an accepting attitude to help increase the patient's feelings of self-worth and emotional security.

34. B: While antidepressants, anticonvulsants, opioids, and amphetamines may trigger psychotic or manic responses, corticosteroids are most likely to do so. A psychotic or manic response is most common after high doses ($\geq$40 mg) of steroid drugs. Symptoms often occur within a few days of onset of therapy with reactions including hypomania, psychosis, and mania. Corticosteroid-induced psychiatric responses are more common in females than males. If symptoms occur, the medication dosage should be tapered to a lower dose and discontinued if possible.

35. C: The most common co-morbid condition of adolescents with bipolar disorder is ADHD. The treatment for ADHD, which often includes stimulants, may exacerbate manic symptoms of bipolar disease, so patients should be treated with mood stabilizers (such as lithium) and stabilized before treatment for ADHD is instituted. Non-stimulant treatments for ADHD, such as bupropion and tricyclic antidepressants may also result in mood swings. ADHD is also common in adults, with about 20% of adults with ADHD having bipolar disorder.

36. C: The most appropriate response to a patient experiencing a sudden panic attack is to stay with the patient and offer reassurance of safety, speaking in a calm and non-threatening manner. Reducing stimuli (noise, light, people) in the immediate area may help to reduce the patient's fears. Once the patient has regained control and the panic attack subsides, the psychiatric and mental health nurse should explore with the patient the cause of the attack to help the patient recognize precipitating factors.

37. B: Patients with borderline personality disorder often experience splitting because they swing from one extreme to another and cannot deal effectively with both negative and positive feelings, so when the patient feels "abandoned" by the nurse whom the patient had previously idealized, the patient recognizes only the negative feelings. Other characteristics include manipulation (to prevent separation anxiety), clinging/distancing (alternating between excessive closeness and discomfort with closeness), self-destructiveness (self-mutilation, suicide), and impulsivity (substance abuse, gambling, promiscuity).

38. A: The most appropriate method of dealing with manipulative and other inappropriate behavior with a patient with bipolar disorder is to use positive reinforcement when the patient exhibits appropriate behavior and negative consequences when the patient exhibits inappropriate behavior. The patient should be apprised of the negative consequences that the patient may incur, and

expectations about behavior should be clearly outlined. The healthcare staff must all be very consistent in applying positive reinforcement and negative consequences.

39. B: An adult can refuse food and nutrition, but a 16-year-old is a minor and under parental control, so the parents/caregivers make the decisions about health. In this case, because the patient's life is in danger, the nurse should respond with what is true and necessary: "You will be fed by nasogastric tube if you don't eat." The patient should be monitored during meals and for at least an hour after meals to prevent purging. A goal for weight gain (usually 2 to 3 pounds per week) should be established and calories/nutrition calculated based on that goal.

40. A: A "state of optimum anxiety" refers to readiness for learning. Studies have indicated that learning is best achieved when the patient is experiencing mild to moderate anxiety, which may be related to anticipation or concerns about learning. This optimum anxiety enhances the ability to concentrate and process information. However, when this level of anxiety is exceeded, learning is impaired and the patient becomes defensive. The psychiatric and mental health nurse may need to assist the patient with anxiety-reducing techniques before teaching.

41. D: The primary focus of the Wellness Recovery Action Plan (WRAP) for group intervention is to help patients to identify personal wellness tools (personal resources) and then to utilize those tools to develop a plan to use when situations arise that threaten the person's health or wellbeing, such as the desire to take drugs or go off of medications. Part of WRAP is to develop a daily maintenance plan and to identify negative triggers and warning signs. The patient identifies what happens when things go very wrong and develops a crisis plan/advance directive and a post-crisis plan.

42. C: Assertive Community Treatment (ACT) is a comprehensive interdisciplinary case-management approach to providing treatment for patients with severe and persistent mental illness. ACT provides services from psychiatry, nursing, social work, and rehabilitation (substance abuse, vocational) around the clock to help patients:
- Decrease/eliminate symptoms
- Minimize recurrent/acute exacerbations
- Meet basic needs
- Improve functioning (social, vocational)
- Live independently

Another goal of the program is to help relieve family members of the burden of caring for patients with serious mental illnesses.

43. D: The most likely reason that Asian-American parents would insist that their child's condition was caused by an "infection" and refuse outpatient care or follow-up is because they are ashamed that their child has a psychiatric condition. It is common among Asian cultures to believe that psychiatric illness is caused by poor behavior, and this behavior is viewed as bringing shame on the patient and the family. Asians often ascribe psychiatric symptoms to physical illnesses, such as infection, because these types of illnesses are more socially acceptable.

44. A: Intellectual disabilities:
- Mild (IQ 60-70): Achieves academic skills to sixth-grade level and is able to learn some vocational skills and to live independently with some assistance.
- Moderate (IQ 35-49): Achieves academic skills to second-grade level and may be able to work in a sheltered workshop, but requires supervision in living situations.

- Severe (IQ 20-34): Learns through systematic habit forming, but cannot benefit from vocational training or work or live independently.
- Profound (IQ <20): Responds to minimal training in self-help and needs constant care and supervision.

45. C: **Secondary preventive measure:** Screening groups that are already identified as at risk for depression, such as older adults, or treating those already diagnosed. These measures typically aim to prevent further deterioration or long-term disease progression. **Primary preventive measures:** Include public service campaigns to educate the general public about depression. These measures aim to reach large numbers of the population. **Tertiary preventive measures:** Includes support groups for patients with depression. These measures aim at management.

46. D: The priority intervention for a patient who presents with multiple injuries is to provide wound care and assess the degree of injury; especially since a head injury is involved. Once the patient's condition is stable, the psychiatric and mental health nurse should ask the patient if she wants to call the police and provide information about domestic abuse services and women's shelters. The nurse should also ascertain that the abuser is not present in the facility because, if that is the case, then security should be notified.

47. B: Safety issues should take priority over others, so the first priority is dealing with the patient's risk for other-directed violence with the short-term goal of the patient discussing feelings and situations that lead to hostility, and the short- and long-term goal of not harming others. The psychiatric and mental health nurse should show an accepting attitude, decrease stimuli, remove all dangerous objects from the patient's environment, and monitor the patient frequently, encouraging the patient to express feelings and explore alternatives to violence while ensuring adequate numbers of staff are present.

48. B: The cycle of battering:
- Phase I, Tension-building: During this state, the abused typically becomes very compliant, trying to defuse the abuser's anger.
- Phase II, Acute battering: The abused typically tries to hide or get away from the abuser. In some cases, the tension from phase I is so severe that the abused may provoke the beating to get it over with.
- Phase III, Respite, loving: The abused feels guilty that the abuser was forced to act and wants to believe that the abuser will remain loving and kind.

49. D: Patients usually exhibit symptoms of abrupt withdrawal from nicotine within 24 hours. Symptoms can include difficulty concentrating, dysphoric or depressed mood, difficulty sleeping, agitation, irritation, anger, frustration, bradycardia, and increased appetite. These symptoms may add to those the patient is already experiencing, making treatment more difficult; so the patient may benefit from the use of nicotine patches to avoid withdrawal symptoms.

50. C: Because the patient does not always seem to understand the questions, this could indicate that the patient is experiencing distortion of sounds related to sensorineural hearing loss, especially since the patient is also speaking in an inappropriately loud tone of voice. This often is a sign of sensorineural hearing loss because the patient is unable to adequately hear his own voice and thus tends to speak loudly to compensate. Additionally, sensorineural hearing loss is most common in older adults.

51. C: An appropriate outcome criterion for a nursing diagnosis of *chronic low self-esteem* is "Patient can verbalize positive self-characteristics." Substance abusers often have longstanding low self-esteem, characterized by lack of eye contact, social isolation, repeatedly failing because of unrealistic goals, projection, lack of responsibility, rationalization, and hypersensitivity to criticism along with the inability to accept positive reinforcement. Goals include the patient's being able to accept personal responsibility for behavior and to exhibit increased feelings of self-worth.

52. B: Because the recovery model maintains focus on the desires of the patient and allows the patient to make decisions, the best approach for the psychiatric and mental health nurse to a patient who plans to stop taking medication is to educate the patient about the needs of the medication and potential outcomes for failing to take the medication. However, adults—unless court-ordered—cannot be forced to take medications, regardless of the extent of their mental illness.

53. D: Even patients who are essentially non-verbal with autism spectrum disorder have usually developed some methods of communication—such as becoming agitated or using random words or gestures—and the best people to understand the way the patient communicates are often the parents or caregivers. These people have spent extensive periods of time with the patient, so the psychiatric and mental health nurse should interview the parents/caregivers about communication strategies in order to have a better understanding of the patient's reactions and methods of communication.

54. A: Sensory stimulation therapy (SST) is based on the concept of neural plasticity and aims to make new connections in the brain to compensate for loss. One type of SST uses items found in a patient's everyday life to stimulate one or more of the five senses. For example, a patient may be asked to smell a particular food and then be asked questions about the food. Another type of SST uses a rapid sequence of nerve stimulation through a device in a part of the body, such as an arm, to promote neural regeneration.

55. C: While there is no evidence that aromatherapy can cure anxiety, some people find aromatherapy relaxing, and this relaxation can help to relieve anxiety. The most appropriate response is" The aromatherapy may help you to relax" because this is true, but does not advocate for or against the therapy. Aromatherapy is essentially benign in that it is neither invasive nor toxic. Aromatherapy is often combined with massage with the essential oils applied directly to the skin, rather than inhaled.

56. A. In psychodrama, the role of the *protagonist* is assumed by the patient who has a problem to resolve. Other members of the therapeutic group assume roles to act out with the protagonist. For example, if a patient has a conflict with a spouse and cannot confront the spouse, a member of a group may act out the role of the spouse. The group leader, usually a therapist or nurse, is referred to as the director and the members of the group, the audience. Participants are actors.

57. B: The patient is exhibiting symptoms of *delirium tremens*, which usually occurs within three to ten days of drinking cessation. The treatment of choice is usually a long-acting benzodiazepine, such as diazepam or lorazepam, to prevent seizures. Phenobarbital may be used as an adjunct but poses more risk of respiratory depression and low blood pressure, although a single dose is sometimes given in the emergency department before the benzodiazepine. If DTs are intractable to benzodiazepine, phenobarbital or propofol may be added.

58. D: Because of enzyme deficiencies that decrease the rate of metabolism for some drugs, Asians (especially Japanese and Chinese) may require lower dosages of benzodiazepines and tricyclic antidepressants. For example, about 20% of Asians metabolize diazepam poorly, so the drug begins to rapidly accumulate and can result in toxic reactions and overdose. Asian patients should be started on low dosages of these drugs and observed carefully. Additionally, some Mexican Americans with variant genes respond better to some antidepressants than those without the variant genes.

59. C: Benzodiazepines are the most-commonly prescribed treatment for generalized anxiety disorder because they are relatively safe, have few drug-drug interactions, and rarely alter consciousness. Commonly used drugs include diazepam, lorazepam, alprazolam, and clonazepam. Benzodiazepines are contraindicated for patients who are pregnant or who have narrow-angle glaucoma. Adverse effects include sedation, hypotension, nausea, vomiting, pruritis, skin rash, and blood dyscrasias (anemia, leukopenia, and thrombocytopenia). Overdose of benzodiazepines may result in severe life-threatening toxicity. Treatment is usually supportive although the antidote, flumazenil, may be used in severe cases.

60. A: When developing a plan of care for an OCD patient who compulsively washes his hands, the first goal in assisting the patient to reduce this ritualistic behavior and to increase coping skills is to assist the patient to recognize precipitating factors. The patient should begin to understand the type of circumstances that serve as triggers. Trying to abruptly stop ritualistic behavior before the patient has developed adequate coping skills may result in extreme anxiety and panic attacks.

61. B: With milieu therapy, all aspects of the patient's environment are considered therapeutic, and patients are expected to be active participants in planning their own treatment. Criteria for milieu therapy include fulfilling basic physiological needs, establishing an environment that is conducive to achieving therapeutic goals, and creating a democratic form of governance in which the patients and staff are equal members and participants. Patients and staff meet in weekly community meetings in order to establish rules, norms, and behavioral expectations and limitations.

62. D: When using cognitive behavioral therapy for treatment of mood disorders, the focus is on changing automatic thoughts or thought distortions. Automatic thoughts related to depression include personalizing, all-or-nothing thinking, mind reading, and discounting positives, while automatic thoughts related to mania include the same type of thoughts except that mania involves discounting negatives. Patients' thought processes are challenged and the affected patient is asked to describe evidence for beliefs. Another approach is to help the patient evaluate what would happen if the automatic thoughts were realistic.

63. A: In the initial period when the patient's medication dosage is being adjusted, the patient should be assisted with ambulation because the patient is at increased risk of falls because of the hypotensive effects of the drug. The patient should be cautioned to sit up slowly and to stay seated for a moment before standing to reduce orthostatic hypotension. The patient's white blood cell count should also be monitored, as this drug may cause leukopenia as well as increased glucose levels and liver enzymes.

64. B: A patient taking clozapine for treatment should be regularly monitored for leukopenia and agranulocytosis with regular WBC counts. Clozapine is recommended for patients with schizophrenia not responding to other treatments and who are at risk for suicide. Clozapine has significant adverse effects, including seizures, cardiomyopathy, myocarditis, pulmonary embolism, and cardiac arrest. The drug should be used with caution with benzodiazepines and other

psychotropic drugs because the combination may result in respiratory arrest. Clozapine has multiple drug-drug interactions so all medications should be carefully reviewed before beginning treatment.

65. C: The action that is most likely to be effective in establishing a relationship of trust with a newly admitted patient is explaining the reason for unit procedures. While routine care—administering medications, providing a list of rules, and giving a tour—may be done in such a caring manner as to engender trust, those things that are "extra," such as taking time to explain procedures, keeping one's word, providing needed food or supplies, considering the patient's preferences, and ensuring confidentiality, are more likely to cause the patient to have confidence and trust in the psychiatric and mental health nurse.

66. D: Sharing personal information, such as by telling about breaking up with a fiancé, is almost always a boundary violation unless it serves a real therapeutic purpose. Even then, self-disclosure should be done judiciously. Finding a patient attractive is not a concern unless the nurse acts on the attraction. Touch is a sensitive issue and can be easily misconstrued, but holding a patient's hand or touching an arm to comfort a patient is usually acceptable. Gifts generally should not be accepted, although candy to be shared with the entire staff is usually an exception.

67. B: While patients may vary in how they express feelings, walking or sitting slumped over, keeping the eyes and head down, avoiding eye contact, failing to initiate conversations, and keeping a low tone of voice are consistent with low self-esteem. The psychiatric and mental health nurse should help the patient to establish realistic and achievable goals and help the patient identify positive personal aspects and strengths. The patient may need one-on-one support in difficult situations, such as group therapy, to deal with fear of failure.

68. C: The most appropriate response to a patient who is pacing and agitated is to describe the behavior observed: "I notice you are pacing and seem upset." The nurse should avoid appearing judgmental or asking "why" but should make the observation and allow the patient to respond, as this helps the patient to recognize behaviors. The nurse should also avoid being directive, such as with "Take a moment and calm down before we proceed," unless a patient's actions are endangering.

69. B: An empathic response is one that shows that the psychiatric and mental health nurse understands what the patient is feeling regardless of outward behavior: "You feel angry and sad about the other patients making fun of you." Empathy is critical to a therapeutic relationship because it helps the patient to identify personal feelings that may be repressed and helps the patient believe the nurse is understanding and caring.

70. A: The therapeutic relationship:
- Pre-interaction: The nurse obtains information about the patient from various sources and examines personal feelings about working with the patient.
- Orientation: The patient and nurse get to know each other, establish rapport, and develop a plan of action based on the patient's strengths and weaknesses and nursing diagnoses.
- Working: The nurse helps the patient engage in problem solving activities and to overcome resistant behaviors, evaluating progress toward goals.
- Termination: The nurse and patient should explore feelings about termination and plan for continuing care.

71. B: When a psychiatric and mental health nurse has difficulty setting limits on a patient's behavior because of an emotional response to a patient, this is an example of **counter transference,** which refers to the emotional response the psychiatric and mental health nurse has toward the patient. **Transference** occurs when the patient transfers feelings and behavior that had been directed toward another person toward the nurse. For example, if the patient hates his mother and the nurse makes a comment that reminds him of her, the patient may transfer his negative feelings toward the nurse.

72. A: Non-therapeutic communication includes inappropriately giving reassurance: "I don't think you need to worry about that." This response suggests that the patient doesn't need to be concerned and devalues what the patient is feeling. This type of response may make the patient reluctant to share feelings in the future. Other types of non-therapeutic communication techniques include rejecting, approving/disapproving, agreeing/disagreeing, giving advice, persistent questioning, defending, asking for explanations, belittling, making stereotypical comments, and changing the subject.

73. A: Feedback that is descriptive and focused on behavior is "Mary was upset and sad when you called her 'stupid and ugly.'" This statement described the action and the result without being evaluative ("mean and rude") or focusing on the patient ("How would you feel...?"). Using evaluative comments often results in the patient becoming defensive. Feedback should be specific and should address things that the patient can actually modify, such as behavior. Feedback should give information rather than advice ("You should apologize..."), and should be given promptly.

74. D: A patient experiencing a severe emotional crisis after her only child leaves home for college is undergoing a crisis of anticipated life transition, which involves a situation that the patient can anticipate and plan for but over which the patient may feel powerless and out of control. Other types of crises include maturational/developmental, dispositional, traumatic stress-related, and psychopathology-related. Patients experiencing a crisis are often not able to problem solve and need support and assistance in order to resolve the crisis.

75. B: The four-phase intervention method (Aguilera, 1998):
   I.   Assessment: Gather information about precipitating factors, events, coping methods, support systems, substance abuse, suicide/homicide potential, and the patient's perceptions of strengths. Develop nursing diagnoses.
   II. Planning intervention: Select actions for nursing diagnoses.
   III. Intervention: Carry out actions, including establishing rapport, setting behavioral limits, clarifying problems, acknowledging feelings, guiding the patient through problem solving, and helping the patient identify new coping mechanisms.
   IV. Evaluation/Anticipatory planning: Evaluate resolution of crisis and discuss how the patient will deal with triggering events in the future.

76. C: About 30 minutes before electroconvulsive therapy (ECT), the patient usually receives a cholinergic blocking agent, such as atropine sulfate or glycopyrrolate, to decrease secretions, reduce the risk of aspiration, and to increase the heart rate to compensate for the slowing that results from vagal stimulation during ECT. During the procedure, the patient usually receives a short-acting anesthetic (such as methohexital sodium) and a muscle relaxant (succinylcholine chloride).

77. A: Before confronting a patient who is at risk for violence, the psychiatric and mental health nurse should first ensure that adequate staff are available to assist and the nurse should alert them

to the situation. The next step is to attempt to talk the patient down. The nurse may suggest physical outlets of aggression (hitting a pillow). The nurse should ask if the patient is willing to take medication voluntarily and should assess if the situation requires medical or mechanical restraints. The patient should be secluded from other patients by taking the patient to a separate area or removing other patients to ensure their safety.

78. B: Patients recovering from electroconvulsive therapy (ECT) usually experience confusion and temporary impairment of memory. Patients should be advised of this before the procedure but may still be quite frightened by this confusion on awakening after ECT. The nurse should provide reassurance, explaining to the patient what has happened and reorienting the patient to time and place. The patient may require very structured activities for a few days after the treatment until memory improves.

79. D: **Projection** occurs when a patient attributes unacceptable personal feelings or behavior to someone else, such as a patient flirting with a nurse and then claiming the nurse was "coming on" to her. **Sublimation** occurs when a patient refocuses unacceptable drives, feelings, or impulses onto something acceptable. **Suppression** occurs when a patient voluntarily blocks or suppresses unpleasant feelings or memories from awareness. **Displacement** occurs when a patient transfers feelings from one person or thing to another that is less threatening.

80. B: A patient's making inappropriate and even threatening comments is not unusual, and the psychiatric and mental health nurse should document this in the nursing notes by reporting exactly what the patient said and the circumstances in which it occurred. If the nurse actually feels threatened, then the issue of safety needs to be addressed by the staff. Whether an incident report needs to be filed depends on the policies of the institution and the degree of threat, and this may require some degree of subjective judgment.

81. C: The statement that suggests that the patient is using the ego defense mechanism of rationalization to explain his throwing a glass of water at the group leader is: "The leader repeatedly egged me on, forcing me to act." This patient is trying to give logical reasons for illogical behavior rather than accepting that his behavior was unacceptable. Ego defense mechanisms are unconscious coping mechanisms that help patients reduce anxiety and are commonly used but become a problem when they affect mental or physical health.

82. A: SAMHSA has many programs aimed at reducing the impact of substance abuse and mental illness. *Opening Doors* is a program aimed at preventing and ending homelessness. The program was developed in 2010 in response to statistics that showed that out of 610,000 homeless people in the United States, about one in five have a serious mental illness and slightly more than one in five are substance abusers. *Opening Doors* helps to ensure collaboration among a number of government agencies, including HHS, Medicaid, and TANF programs.

83. D: Under the Americans with Disabilities Act, employers are under no obligation to provide accommodations for disabling conditions about which they are unaware. Therefore, if the patient wants work accommodations, the patient must disclose that he has a disability. Once the patient has disclosed this information, then the patient is protected by the ADA, and the employer must provide reasonable accommodations as prescribed by law. Employers cannot ask potential or current employees if they have disabilities, but employers can ask if people need accommodations.

84. B: In most states, there is no legal mechanism for requiring compliance with advance directives, and the reality is that, despite these directives, physicians rarely insist on removing life support and

allowing patients to die if family members object. Additionally, "no heroic measures" is a general term that can be interpreted in different ways. In this case, the most appropriate course of action for the psychiatric and mental health nurse is to remain supportive and provide education to the family, who may need time to accept the reality of the patient's condition.

85. C: The Health Insurance Portability and Accountability Act (1996) (HIPAA) protects the confidentiality of medical records and ensures that patients have access to their medical records because, while the originator owns the actual record, the information contained in the record belongs to the patient. HIPAA also gives patients the right to have corrections made in their records if they feel that the records contain errors. Protected health information (PHI) is almost any information that identifies the person.

86. A: The International Society of Psychiatric-Mental Health Nurses (ISPN) states in "Emergency Care Psychiatric Clinical Framework" that the clinical assessment of the patient in the emergency department should begin with a focused medical assessment that is relevant to the psychiatric patient to determine if the patient has a medical condition contributing to the psychiatric symptoms or has a medical condition in addition to the psychiatric symptoms. This should be followed by a psychiatric evaluation that includes a mental status exam.

87. B: The American Nurses Association (ANA) has over 3 million members and is the most active organization politically through its national, state, and local affiliates. The ANA lobbies and promotes legislation related to the needs of the nursing profession and has taken an active role in developing policy initiatives related to healthcare reform. The ANA has taken positions on a number of issues that relate to both nurses and patients in relation to workplace safety and improvement in healthcare delivery.

88. C: The most effective position for active listening is sitting directly in front of the patient with arms and legs uncrossed so that the psychiatric and mental health nurse appears open to the patient's comments. The nurse should lean slightly toward the patient to indicate interest and should establish eye contact, although the eye contact should not be overly aggressive or staring, as this may be intimidating. The nurse should relax and appear comfortable with the patient.

89. D: The initial recommendation should be for respite care to relieve the caregiver of the responsibility for constant care for at least a short period of time. Respite care may be available through various sources, such as Alzheimer's organizations, the Older Americans Act, or hospice. Realistically, family and friends are not always available or willing to assist, and long-term care facilities can be prohibitively expensive unless the patient qualifies for Medicaid. A support group is a good recommendation for ongoing support.

90. A: The Older Americans Act (OAA) (1965, 2006) is intended to improve access to a variety of services for older adults and Native Americans by providing funding to local organizations and agencies. Services include home delivery of meals, transportation, adult day care, home repair, and legal assistance. Programs are also available to combat violence against older adults. The National Family Caregivers Support Act is part of OAA and provides services to caregivers. Services that are available may vary from community to community.

91. B: When a patient thinks, "If I stop drinking, I can repair my marriage," this type of "self-talk" is referred to as **uncertainty reduction** because the patient is going through a thought process to reduce uncertainty about a decision. **Uncertainty maintenance**, however, occurs when thought processes increase or maintain doubt about a decision. **Realistic goal setting** is setting goals that

are reasonably attainable in order to facilitate success. **Learner readiness** involves the desire and willingness to move toward a goal.

92. A: Keller's ARCS model focuses on creating a learning environment that includes motivational strategies to facilitate learning when designing instruction for the learner. The ARCS model comprises:
- Attention: Uses variable instructional methods, opposing positions, participatory discussions.
- Relevance: Utilizes knowledge, choices, and experiences the learner brings to the process.
- Confidence: Considers requirements of learning, difficulty level, goals, attributions, personal sense of accomplishment.
- Satisfaction: Includes reward systems, praise, learner use of new skill and personal evaluation.

93. A: When prioritizing needs, those that are physiological are the priority. In this case, the patient is experiencing both pain and anxiety, and pain usually must be dealt with first, followed by anxiety reduction through relaxation techniques. Anxiety may, in fact, be related to the degree of pain. Dietary instruction is of practical use and should be carried out next. Disease pathology may or may not be of particular interest to a patient, but knowledge of disease pathology is not essential in learning to manage self-care.

94. D: Encoding is the method by which perceptions, feelings, and thoughts are converted into memories. **Elaborative encoding:** Relating new information to knowledge that patients already have in memory. This is one of the most effective methods of encoding. **Organizational encoding:** Organizing or chunking information into groups according to relationships. **Spontaneous/Automatic encoding:** Memory occurring without effort or conscious thought, such as what might occur with an unusual or frightening event. **Visual encoding:** Storing information in memory by converting it into visual images.

95. C: Types of readiness to learn:
- **Experiential:** Includes coping mechanisms, orientation, degree of aspirations, and cultural background.
- **Emotional:** Includes level of anxiety, support systems, motivation, frame of mind, developmental stage, and risk-taking behavior.
- **Physical:** Includes ability, task complexity, health, age, gender, and effects of the environment.
- **Knowledge:** Includes current knowledge base, cognitive ability, learning style, and learning disabilities.

96. A: All video materials prepared for patients should have closed-captioning; this is the most appropriate accommodation, as it allows the patient to participate in the group without drawing attention to the patient's hearing loss. A script should be available for any audio materials. When developing materials, the psychiatric and mental health nurse should always consider the possible need for alternative delivery for patients, especially those with hearing, vision, or cognitive impairment.

97. D: When the psychiatric and mental health nurse is serving as a preceptor for a student, the primary responsibility is teaching and promoting student learning, although the preceptor should maintain contact with the student's clinical instructor and discuss student progress with the

instructor on a regular basis. At the beginning of a preceptorship, the nurse should meet with the student and instructor to discuss expectations and procedures and to facilitate good communication among the three.

98. B: Trust is the key ingredient in developing a learning contract with a patient; the contract should be culturally sensitive and developmentally appropriate. Learning contracts may be formal or informal, but should include goals and a plan of action as well as a method of evaluation. The learning contract should be developed in collaboration with the patient, who trusts the nurse to provide guidance, learning materials, and learning opportunities, and the nurse, who trusts the patient to follow through with the learning contract.

99. A: Illicit drug users should be advised to have vaccinations for hepatitis A and B. Hepatitis A is recommended for those who take illicit drugs by any method and hepatitis B for those who use injection drugs. Hepatitis A is spread by the oral-fecal route. Those most at risk are people having sex with infected persons, travelers to endemic areas, men having sex with men, and illicit drug users. Hepatitis B is spread through contact with an infected person's blood or body fluids, putting injection drug users at special risk, especially from sharing needles.

100. D: When serving as a mentor to a newly hired nurse, the psychiatric and mental health nurse should remain as supportive as possible, helping the person to self-evaluate and learn. The most appropriate response is the one that encourages the nurse to come up with a solution: "How do you think you might have handled that differently?" The mentoring nurse should avoid direct criticism ("You didn't handle that situation well"), negative questioning ("What do you think you did wrong?"), and solutions ("Always call for help").

101. C: The minimum recommended amount of walking or other moderate-intensity aerobic exercises per week is 150 minutes. This can be done in differing amounts per day, but for sufficient cardiovascular benefit, the period of walking should be at least 10 minutes each time. Ideally, patients should walk 30 minutes daily in addition to muscle-building exercises, which are also important. Moderate-intensity exercises include walking, water aerobics, playing tennis (doubles), and riding a bicycle. High-intensity exercises include jogging/running, swimming laps, riding a bicycle fast or over hills, and playing tennis (singles).

102. D: Core principles of peer review include focusing on nursing practice. The peer review should always be done by someone of the same rank and not by a supervisor, as this is a different type of evaluation. Peer review should be carried out on a routine basis with prompt feedback from the reviewer to the reviewee in an open discussion. Peer review should never be carried out anonymously. It should consider the developmental stage of the nurse, so expectations of a newly graduated nurse might be different from those of an experienced nurse, even at the same rank.

103. B: The American Psychiatric Nurses Association (APNA) has taken the position that the use of seclusion and restraints is not supported by research and should be reduced or eliminated and, when used, should be applied with the fewest points of restraint for the shortest necessary time and allow the most freedom of movement possible. The APNA urges that institutions develop evidence-based practices to be utilized during behavioral emergencies and to reduce incidences of aggression and violence.

104. C: Rational coping requires the patient to actively engage a stressor even though it may be painful initially in order to move past the trauma. Rational coping comprises three steps:

- Acceptance: Accepting that the event happened rather than trying to deny or repress the event.
- Exposure: Exposing oneself to the stressor by thinking and talking about it and describing the event so that it loses power.
- Understanding: Making an effort to understand the meaning of the event in the person's life.

105. D: While there is some variation among Native American tribes, generally Native Americans are comfortable with prolonged silences during conversation, so the nurse should resist filling the silence with comments. Native Americans are often uncomfortable with direct eye contact, they like a large personal space separating them from others, and are uncomfortable with being touched. While norms may apply to a cultural group as a whole, the psychiatric and mental health nurse must always remember that the norms may not always apply to the individual.

106. A: Giving tokens as a reward for desired behaviors is an example of positive reinforcement, which is a strategy used in behavioral therapy, which focuses on modifying behavior rather than trying to understand the unconscious motivation for the behavior. Behavioral therapy is based on the premise that inappropriate behavior is learned and can be changed. One disadvantage to this approach is that the learned behavior may only be evident when the reward is being given and does not continue when the reward is removed.

107. C: While there is some value to all of these approaches, the most effective treatment approach for a severe phobia, such as fear of heights, is exposure therapy. This approach reduces fear by gradually exposing the patient to the feared situation or object. This repeated stimulus tends to decrease the emotional response over time. Exposure therapy utilizes an exposure hierarchy in which the patient ranks fears on a continuum so that the patient can be exposed to the least stressful for practice first.

108. B: A patient who changes her perceptions and the way she thinks to allow her to cope with and overcome stressors is utilizing reframing. Reframing can be helpful if the situation is one that the person can think about in advance in order to develop a more creative frame of mind; however, if the event/situation is so stressful that the person cannot bear to even think about it, then this technique is not likely to be effective.

109. D: Patients with antisocial personality disorder may benefit from milieu therapy because the focus is on community and participation with others, allowing the patient to develop social skills. Because the patient resents authority, the person may be more receptive to peer feedback from other patients than from authority figures, such as staff members. The milieu community in many ways mimics social situations the patient must deal with in everyday life, so participating in the development of rules and interacting with others may help the patient recognize appropriate behavior.

110. C: **NAMI** programs:
- **Basics:** Especially designed to provide strategies for caregiving for parents/caregivers of children or adolescents with mental illness.
- **Peer-to-Peer:** Designed for adults with mental illness to provide education and skills needed to prevent relapse, make decisions, interact with healthcare providers, and reduce stress.
- **Family-to-Family:** Designed for family/caregivers of people with mental illness to provide educations and strategies for caregiving.

- **Homefront:** New program designed for family/caregivers of military service members/veterans with mental illness.

111. B: Under the ANA's *Code of Ethics,* if the psychiatric and mental health nurse feels that a research project is morally objectionable, the nurse has the right to question, report, and refuse to participate. When involved in research projects, the nurse should be aware of all legal requirements regarding patient consent and confidentiality, and should ensure that patients understand their right to refuse to participate. The nurse must also be aware of special consideration for protected populations of patients, such as children and prisoners.

112. A: When conducting a community assessment for preventive health measures as part of community-based care, the three primary factors to consider are:
- People: This includes family, friends, and community members who may help support or interfere with preventive health measures.
- Environment: This includes an assessment of the location and its surroundings as well as the domicile to determine if they are likely to support preventive health measures.
- Social systems: This includes assessing which community resources are available and how they may affect preventive health measures.

113. B: Homeless shelters vary considerably; some require people to line up at certain hours to gain access, while others have waiting lists. Finding housing can be overwhelming to some patients, who may find it easier to simply live on the streets. The best plan is for the psychiatric and mental health nurse to contact shelters prior to discharge to try to secure a place for the patient. If that isn't likely, the nurse should get as much information as possible about the process of obtaining shelter so that the patient knows exactly what steps to take.

114. D: While nutritional counseling may be of value, the immediate needs relate to lack of money, so the most appropriate recommendation is to local food banks, which should be able to provide groceries to those with low income. Home delivery of meals is usually restricted to the elderly or disabled and not available to the general public. WIC programs serve mothers up to a year after delivery if breastfeeding and children until their fifth birthday, so this family is no longer eligible.

115. C: Overeaters Anonymous® is a 12-step support group that is focused on helping patients recover from compulsive eating as well as any eating disorder, such as anorexia or bulimia. Because participants often have severe weight problems or eating disorders, a patient who is morbidly obese may feel more comfortable in this group rather than Weight Watchers®, which attracts a different range of participants. Overeaters Anonymous® addresses not only the physical problems associated with compulsive eating but also emotional aspects. It is a peer-led group.

116. B: When interacting with a patient who is vision-impaired, the psychiatric and mental health nurse should explain and describe actions as they are being carried out. The nurse should allow others who are present to introduce themselves so that the patient can hear their voices and identify their locations in the room. Holding the patient's hand is not necessary, but the nurse should announce presence when entering the room or gently touch the patient. While it's not necessary to stand in front of the patient when addressing the patient, the nurse should avoid addressing the patient from behind.

117. C: While the patient should not be imbibing alcohol at all when in a recovery program for cocaine abuse, the patient is participating in sexual activity that places him at high risk for sexually-transmitted diseases; the initial screening should be for STDs so that necessary treatment can be

provided if the patient tests positive. Drug and alcohol abuse is often accompanied by other high-risk activities because of lack of inhibition, poor judgment, and low sense of self-esteem.

118. A: If the patient's insurance plan will not cover the cost of outpatient therapy, then the best alternative when modifying the patient's plan of care is likely a referral to Narcotics Anonymous® (NA), which is a 12-step peer-led support group that helps prevent relapse. There is no cost for participating in NA, and the patient can request a sponsor with whom the patient can communicate concerns and who can serve as a source of support for the patient.

119. B: The normal range for the Q-T interval is 0.36 to 0.44 seconds with the normal for males <0.43 seconds and females <0.45 seconds. Critical measure is ≥0.50 seconds. The Q-T measure varies somewhat from person to person and is longer with a slow pulse than a fast pulse. When monitoring, the psychiatric and mental health nurse should monitor with a lead in which the T wave is clearly evident on the tracing. Q-T prolongation may result from numerous drugs, including amitriptyline, aripiprazole, chlorpromazine, citalopram, olanzapine, quetiapine, sertraline, and methadone.

120. D: While state laws regarding privacy and audio/video recording vary somewhat, generally video monitoring without consent is allowed in all public areas within a unit, such as the recreation room, hallways, and stairwells, although patients should be notified if monitoring is used. Without consent or court order, videotaping of the patient in the bedroom or bathroom is generally prohibited. When utilizing videotaping, the monitors should be placed so that they cannot be viewed by anyone but authorized staff members.

121. A: The most appropriate solution to prevent further falls is to place a pressure-sensitive movement pad with an alarm beneath the patient because this will alert the nursing staff when the patient is no longer reclining. Physical restraints should not be used to prevent falls from beds as they may result in other injuries. Providing a sitter for one patient is expensive, especially on an ongoing basis. Moving the patient's bed to a room next to a nursing desk is a good strategy because the room can be accessed faster, but that alone is not likely to prevent falls.

122. D: When educating a patient about vagus nerve stimulation, it's important for the patient to understand not to expect an immediate response because the positive effects of the treatment occur slowly over a long period of time, up to about 9 months for many patients. Patients should also understand that they should continue with other prescribed treatments for depression. During times of stimulation, patients may experience hoarseness, cough, and/or dyspnea, but symptoms usually subside quickly.

123. B: Serious reportable events (SREs) are those that should be preventable with good practices but that result in severe injury or death: Patient elopes from the hospital and is killed when running into traffic. The National Quality Forum (NQF) first endorsed a list of SREs in 2002 and encourages healthcare providers to report these events. SREs fall into seven categories: surgical/invasive procedures, product or device, patient protection, care management, environmental, radiologic, and potential criminal.

124. C: Providing a concrete plan of action, such as a discharge checklist that is to be utilized with all patients, is more likely to result in variance reduction than using negative or positive reinforcement because that alone provides no guidance regarding what needs to be done to make changes. Quality variance occurs when there is an inconsistency in findings, such as increased

infections in one unit or decreased compliance with follow-up. The initial step in variance reduction is to determine the cause of the variance.

125. C: Symptoms associated with serotonin syndrome include agitation, myoclonus, hyperreflexia, coarse tremors, diaphoresis, tachycardia, confusion, dilated pupils, fever, and diarrhea. More severe life-threatening symptoms include hyperthermia, seizures, rhabdomyolysis, kidney failure, cardiac dysrhythmias, and DIC. Identifying the symptoms and discontinuing the causal drugs usually reverses mild to moderate symptoms. Other treatments include serotonin blocking agents, muscle relaxants; and supportive treatment for elevated BP, pulse rate and dyspnea.

126. A: Hypokalemia (levels <3.5 mEq/L) indicates that the patient has resumed purging, although many patients who are purging have normal levels of potassium, so potassium level alone is not sufficient for evaluation. Electrolyte imbalances may relate to the purging mechanism (vomiting, laxative use, diuretic use). Some patients will show metabolic alkalosis and others metabolic acidosis. Elevated serum amylase and bicarbonate levels often occur with vomiting, although serum bicarbonate levels may decrease with laxative use.

127. D: When a patient is emotionally upset and crying, the best response is to sit quietly with the patient, allowing the patient to express feelings. The nurse should avoid reinforcing guilty feelings the patient may have, as this is not therapeutic; the nurse should also not try to change the patient's focus or the topic of conversation. While hugging may be comforting to some people, physical touch can be misconstrued, especially by patients who are in vulnerable states, so nurses should avoid hugging patients.

128. C: UAP may monitor a patient's intake of food during a meal and may take routine vital signs (such as during each shift), but the UAP may not take the initial vital signs during the admission physical because these are part of the patient assessment and must be done by the nurse. UAPs may check on physical restraints to make sure they are secure and properly in place and may remove them but may not apply the restraints. The UAP may not administer medications.

129. A: When obtaining a history for an adolescent, the psychiatric and mental health nurse should request that the parents/caregivers wait in another area so that the interview can be conducted in private as adolescents are often very reluctant to share personal information with a parent/caregiver present. The psychiatric and mental health nurse should explain that the purpose of the private interview is to help the adolescent begin to assume personal responsibility for health needs and the nurse should ask the parents/caregivers if they have any concerns they want addressed or any questions.

130. B: The statement that "I believe that someone born a man is always a man" is judgmental and suggests that the psychiatric and mental health nurse's attitude may negatively impact delivery of care of the patient, who would expect to be referred to with female pronouns and treated as a woman. Indicating a lack of understanding: "I don't really understand…" and asking about how to address the person shows that the nurse is trying to clarify information in order to better care for the patient. "I try to treat everyone the same…" indicates an openness toward patients.

131. A: The first step in de-escalation of a patient is to remove the other patients from the room to calm the environment. While it is common to call for a team in the early stages of de-escalation, the team should be nearby but not threatening to the patient who may further escalate if the patient feels intimidated. A third party "negotiator" from the team who was not part of the activity that

brought about the escalation may be able to calmly talk the patient down. Restraints should be avoided whenever possible.

132. D: One of the disadvantages of the 15-year-old patient attending a support group is that the patient may be exposed to other patients with more severe symptoms and may pick up negative behaviors because adolescents often emulate others. For example, the patient may learn about taking diuretics for weight loss from discussions in the group. However, the patient may benefit from learning how peers have dealt with similar issues, so the benefits must be weighed against the disadvantages on an individual basis.

133. C: When utilizing Focus Charting for documentation, the focus (problem) may be on current or future patient behavior or concerns, nursing diagnosis (but not medical diagnosis), change in patient's behavior/status, or an important event/change related to the patient's therapy. Documentation is organized into three columns, using the DAR approach for progress notes:
1. Date and time
2. Focus problem
3. Progress note: **Data** regarding the stated focus, **action** to address the focus, and **response** to action

134. B: When a patient is suicidal, the most important consideration is that the patient not be left alone. Someone should agree to stay with the patient or the patient should stay with family or friends. Additionally, the patient should be asked to sign a no-suicide contract, and family or friends should remove dangerous items, such as knives, from the patient's home. Appointments for follow-up (daily at first) should be made prior to discharge, and the psychiatric and mental health nurse should speak directly to the patient about suicide plans.

135. D: Since the area of the form for "current medications" was left blank, the psychiatric and mental health nurse should contact the board and care facility to verify this information because the transfer form should have included a notation of "no medications." The patient may not be reliable since he is experiencing a psychotic episode, and the psychiatrist may not be aware of medications or treatments the patient may have received from other physicians.

136. A: While Medicare does cover home health care for patients over 65, these patients must meet eligibility requirements. One primary requirement is that the patient be essentially homebound, so the patient's "debilitating physical condition that makes travel difficult" may make the patient eligible. Lack of transportation or simple desire not to waste time traveling is not a criterion to justify home health care. Most communities have transportation available for those who are over 65 with health problems.

137. B: The three components of panic control treatment (PCT), which is a form of cognitive behavioral therapy that focuses on reducing the patient's anxiety about having a panic attack, include:
- Cognitive restructuring: Patient is helped to explore physical response realistically in order to recognize that physical damage is not occurring.
- *In vivo* exposure: Patient is systematically exposed to the thing that causes the panic attack to reduce the response.
- Interoceptive exposure: Patient induces panic-like responses, such as through hyperventilation, to begin desensitization.

138. A: **Hamilton Anxiety Rating Scale:** Used to evaluate the level and severity of anxiety in adults and children. May be utilized for drug evaluation at the beginning of treatment with anti-anxiety drugs and during treatment to adjust dosage and determine outcomes. **Psychological Screening Inventory:** Used for adults and adolescents to assess psychological status to determine the need for psychological treatment. **Milton Clinical Multiaxial Inventory:** Used to assess personality and psychopathology. **Beck Anxiety Inventory:** Used to assess anxiety as low, moderate, or severe.

139. A: Conversion disorders mimic neurological impairment but are caused by psychological factors. Patients characteristically exhibit *la belle indifference,* appearing unconcerned about the symptoms. Onset is typically sudden and corresponds to the degree of knowledge the patient has about the mimicked disorder. The less education the patient has about the disorder, the more atypical and extreme the symptoms. Symptoms may, for example, follow a pattern that doesn't exist in a real disorder. Patients tend to have low education and low socioeconomic status.

140. D: Habit reversal therapy (HRT) steps:
- Awareness: Keeping a behavior log to recognize unconscious behaviors, including emotional states associated with the behavior.
- Trigger identification: Identifying things that trigger the urge.
- Assessment: Identifying negative and positive feelings associated with the behavior.
- Competitive response: Carrying out a competing action to prevent the behavior, such as tapping the wrist rather than pulling hair.
- Assessment of rationalizations: Recognizing rationalizations used to continue the behavior.
- Mindfulness: Controlling urges through understanding and awareness.

141. D: The focus of Acceptance Commitment Therapy (ACT), which is a form of behavioral therapy, is on the patient's examining thought processes through *cognitive defusion* during an anxiety attack. The patient identifies the negative thought and then compiles a list of evidence to determine if the thought has a basis in fact. The patient may do this manually in the beginning but automatically later. The basic steps involved in ACT are (A) acceptance, (C) choosing, and (T) taking action.

142. C: Determination. Motivation Enhancement Therapy (MET) is a non-confrontational approach to behavior modification usually done in 4 meetings and involving six stages:
- Pre-contemplation: Patient is not motivated to change behavior.
- Contemplation: Patient begins to consider the negative and positive aspects of substance abuse.
- Determination: Patient decides to change behavior and stop using.
- Action: Patient takes steps to modify behavior over a period of time.
- Maintenance: Patient stays abstinent.
- Relapse: Patient begins using and then starts the cycle of stages again. Most patients go through a number of relapses.

143. B: Psychological factors:
- **Resourcefulness:** Using problem-solving skills, such as health-seeking strategies, and coping strategies to deal with stressful situations, such as illness, without developing stress.
- **Resilience:** Having the ability to cope with stress and not be overwhelmed.
- **Self-efficacy:** Having the belief that the events in life are affected by behavior and having high motivation and setting high personal goals.
- **Hardiness:** Having the ability to deal with stress without developing illness and to grow from the experience of stress.

144. A: Because therapy should remain focused on the patient, progress should be as well. The most appropriate feedback is a factual observation: "I noticed you were sitting with other patients during the concert." This allows the patient to reflect on the activity without the psychiatric and mental health nurse applying a value judgment, such as "I was so happy..." or "Sitting with other patients is a good sign...". The nurse should avoid questioning the patient about the reasons for a change in behavior, "Why did you...?".

145. A: Patients undergoing acute withdrawal from opioids typically exhibit hypertension and tachycardia as well as piloerection, diaphoresis, rhinorrhea, diarrhea, muscle cramps, arthralgia, nausea, vomiting, anxiety, and lethargy. The peak period for symptoms is one to three days after cessation with symptoms lasing for five to seven days. Medications used for treatment of opioid withdrawal include clonidine or methadone. Naltrexone is sometimes used to block opioid receptors so that the drug does not produce euphoria, but the patient must be without symptoms of withdrawal for at least a week before naltrexone is started.

146. B: These symptoms are consistent with acetaldehyde syndrome, which occurs if a patient who is taking disulfiram ingests even 7 mL of alcohol. Because the symptoms began shortly after the friend left, the most likely cause is that the friend gave the patient alcohol. Disulfiram alters the metabolism of alcohol so that blood levels rise precipitously within 5 to 10 minutes. The symptoms usually begin to recede within about 30 minutes, but some may persist for several hours.

147. D: Foods that are aged are high in tyramine, so patients taking MAO inhibitors should be advised to avoid foods such as aged cheeses or sour products, such as buttermilk, yogurt, and sour cream. Other foods to avoid include bananas, overripe fruits, chocolate, canned meats, dried meats, salami, alcoholic beverages, soy sauce, MSG, yeast concentrates, and packaged soups. Combining these foods with an MAO inhibitor may result in life-threatening hypertensive crisis. Symptoms can include hypertension, palpitations/tachycardia, headache, nuchal rigidity, nausea, and vomiting.

148. C: The nursing diagnosis that is appropriate for the patient's ritualistic and obsessive thoughts is *ineffective coping.* The outcome criteria are that the patient will be able to demonstrate effective coping without resorting to the ritualistic behavior and obsessive thoughts. At the onset of treatment, the patient should be allowed to complete rituals, but the patient should try to identify stressors that trigger the behavior and should, over time, require less time for the behavior as the patient replaces the behavior with more adaptive behavior.

149. B: The woman is undergoing a common response in the aftermath of a disaster. The most appropriate response is to provide support, reassure the woman, and discuss the normal stages of grief and associated feelings. While it's good to reassure the woman that she is safe, platitudes such as "everything will be all right," should be avoided. Anti-anxiety medication is only indicated if the symptoms of anxiety persist for an extended period. Family and friends may not be readily available.

150. D: One of the most important goals of family-focused psychoeducational (FFP) treatment for bipolar disorder is for family members to learn to recognize early warning signs of relapse. FFP should help improve communication between the patient and family members provide information about symptoms, etiology, treatment, and management of the disorder, including medications and adverse effects. Family members should be made aware that at least some of the patient's inappropriate behaviors can be attributed to the disorder.

Secret Key #1 - Time is Your Greatest Enemy

Pace Yourself

Wear a watch. At the beginning of the test, check the time (or start a chronometer on your watch to count the minutes), and check the time after every few questions to make sure you are "on schedule."

If you are forced to speed up, do it efficiently. Usually one or more answer choices can be eliminated without too much difficulty. Above all, don't panic. Don't speed up and just begin guessing at random choices. By pacing yourself, and continually monitoring your progress against your watch, you will always know exactly how far ahead or behind you are with your available time. If you find that you are one minute behind on the test, don't skip one question without spending any time on it, just to catch back up. Take 15 fewer seconds on the next four questions, and after four questions you'll have caught back up. Once you catch back up, you can continue working each problem at your normal pace.

Furthermore, don't dwell on the problems that you were rushed on. If a problem was taking up too much time and you made a hurried guess, it must be difficult. The difficult questions are the ones you are most likely to miss anyway, so it isn't a big loss. It is better to end with more time than you need than to run out of time.

Lastly, sometimes it is beneficial to slow down if you are constantly getting ahead of time. You are always more likely to catch a careless mistake by working more slowly than quickly, and among very high-scoring test takers (those who are likely to have lots of time left over), careless errors affect the score more than mastery of material.

Secret Key #2 - Guessing is not Guesswork

You probably know that guessing is a good idea - unlike other standardized tests, there is no penalty for getting a wrong answer. Even if you have no idea about a question, you still have a 20-25% chance of getting it right.

Most test takers do not understand the impact that proper guessing can have on their score. Unless you score extremely high, guessing will significantly contribute to your final score.

Monkeys Take the Test

What most test takers don't realize is that to insure that 20-25% chance, you have to guess randomly. If you put 20 monkeys in a room to take this test, assuming they answered once per question and behaved themselves, on average they would get 20-25% of the questions correct. Put 20 test takers in the room, and the average will be much lower among guessed questions. Why?

1. The test writers intentionally writes deceptive answer choices that "look" right. A test taker has no idea about a question, so picks the "best looking" answer, which is often wrong. The monkey has no idea what looks good and what doesn't, so will consistently be lucky about 20-25% of the time.
2. Test takers will eliminate answer choices from the guessing pool based on a hunch or intuition. Simple but correct answers often get excluded, leaving a 0% chance of being correct. The monkey has no clue, and often gets lucky with the best choice.

This is why the process of elimination endorsed by most test courses is flawed and detrimental to your performance- test takers don't guess, they make an ignorant stab in the dark that is usually worse than random.

$5 Challenge

Let me introduce one of the most valuable ideas of this course- the $5 challenge:

You only mark your "best guess" if you are willing to bet $5 on it.
You only eliminate choices from guessing if you are willing to bet $5 on it.

Why $5? Five dollars is an amount of money that is small yet not insignificant, and can really add up fast (20 questions could cost you $100). Likewise, each answer choice on one question of the test will have a small impact on your overall score, but it can really add up to a lot of points in the end.

The process of elimination IS valuable. The following shows your chance of guessing it right:

If you eliminate wrong answer choices until only this many remain:	1	2	3
Chance of getting it correct:	100%	50%	33%

However, if you accidentally eliminate the right answer or go on a hunch for an incorrect answer, your chances drop dramatically: to 0%. By guessing among all the answer choices, you are GUARANTEED to have a shot at the right answer.

That's why the $5 test is so valuable- if you give up the advantage and safety of a pure guess, it had better be worth the risk.

What we still haven't covered is how to be sure that whatever guess you make is truly random. Here's the easiest way:

Always pick the first answer choice among those remaining.

Such a technique means that you have decided, **before you see a single test question**, exactly how you are going to guess- and since the order of choices tells you nothing about which one is correct, this guessing technique is perfectly random.

This section is not meant to scare you away from making educated guesses or eliminating choices- you just need to define when a choice is worth eliminating. The $5 test, along with a pre-defined random guessing strategy, is the best way to make sure you reap all of the benefits of guessing.

Secret Key #3 - Practice Smarter, Not Harder

Many test takers delay the test preparation process because they dread the awful amounts of practice time they think necessary to succeed on the test. We have refined an effective method that will take you only a fraction of the time.

There are a number of "obstacles" in your way to succeed. Among these are answering questions, finishing in time, and mastering test-taking strategies. All must be executed on the day of the test at peak performance, or your score will suffer. The test is a mental marathon that has a large impact on your future.

Just like a marathon runner, it is important to work your way up to the full challenge. So first you just worry about questions, and then time, and finally strategy:

Success Strategy

1. Find a good source for practice tests.
2. If you are willing to make a larger time investment, consider using more than one study guide- often the different approaches of multiple authors will help you "get" difficult concepts.
3. Take a practice test with no time constraints, with all study helps "open book." Take your time with questions and focus on applying strategies.
4. Take a practice test with time constraints, with all guides "open book."
5. Take a final practice test with no open material and time limits

If you have time to take more practice tests, just repeat step 5. By gradually exposing yourself to the full rigors of the test environment, you will condition your mind to the stress of test day and maximize your success.

Secret Key #4 - Prepare, Don't Procrastinate

Let me state an obvious fact: if you take the test three times, you will get three different scores. This is due to the way you feel on test day, the level of preparedness you have, and, despite the test writers' claims to the contrary, some tests WILL be easier for you than others.

Since your future depends so much on your score, you should maximize your chances of success. In order to maximize the likelihood of success, you've got to prepare in advance. This means taking practice tests and spending time learning the information and test taking strategies you will need to succeed.

Never take the test as a "practice" test, expecting that you can just take it again if you need to. Feel free to take sample tests on your own, but when you go to take the official test, be prepared, be focused, and do your best the first time!

Secret Key #5 - Test Yourself

Everyone knows that time is money. There is no need to spend too much of your time or too little of your time preparing for the test. You should only spend as much of your precious time preparing as is necessary for you to get the score you need.

Once you have taken a practice test under real conditions of time constraints, then you will know if you are ready for the test or not.

If you have scored extremely high the first time that you take the practice test, then there is not much point in spending countless hours studying. You are already there.

Benchmark your abilities by retaking practice tests and seeing how much you have improved. Once you score high enough to guarantee success, then you are ready.

If you have scored well below where you need, then knuckle down and begin studying in earnest. Check your improvement regularly through the use of practice tests under real conditions. Above all, don't worry, panic, or give up. The key is perseverance!

Then, when you go to take the test, remain confident and remember how well you did on the practice tests. If you can score high enough on a practice test, then you can do the same on the real thing.

General Strategies

The most important thing you can do is to ignore your fears and jump into the test immediately- do not be overwhelmed by any strange-sounding terms. You have to jump into the test like jumping into a pool- all at once is the easiest way.

Make Predictions

As you read and understand the question, try to guess what the answer will be. Remember that several of the answer choices are wrong, and once you begin reading them, your mind will immediately become cluttered with answer choices designed to throw you off. Your mind is typically the most focused immediately after you have read the question and digested its contents. If you can, try to predict what the correct answer will be. You may be surprised at what you can predict.

Quickly scan the choices and see if your prediction is in the listed answer choices. If it is, then you can be quite confident that you have the right answer. It still won't hurt to check the other answer choices, but most of the time, you've got it!

Answer the Question

It may seem obvious to only pick answer choices that answer the question, but the test writers can create some excellent answer choices that are wrong. Don't pick an answer just because it sounds right, or you believe it to be true. It MUST answer the question. Once you've made your selection, always go back and check it against the question and make sure that you didn't misread the question, and the answer choice does answer the question posed.

Benchmark

After you read the first answer choice, decide if you think it sounds correct or not. If it doesn't, move on to the next answer choice. If it does, mentally mark that answer choice. This doesn't mean that you've definitely selected it as your answer choice, it just means that it's the best you've seen thus far. Go ahead and read the next choice. If the next choice is worse than the one you've already selected, keep going to the next answer choice. If the next choice is better than the choice you've already selected, mentally mark the new answer choice as your best guess.
The first answer choice that you select becomes your standard. Every other answer choice must be benchmarked against that standard. That choice is correct until proven otherwise by another answer choice beating it out. Once you've decided that no other answer choice seems as good, do one final check to ensure that your answer choice answers the question posed.

Valid Information

Don't discount any of the information provided in the question. Every piece of information may be necessary to determine the correct answer. None of the information in the question is there to throw you off (while the answer choices will certainly have information to throw you off). If two seemingly unrelated topics are discussed, don't ignore either. You can be confident there is a relationship, or it wouldn't be included in the question, and you are probably going to have to determine what is that relationship to find the answer.

Avoid "Fact Traps"

Don't get distracted by a choice that is factually true. Your search is for the answer that answers the question. Stay focused and don't fall for an answer that is true but incorrect. Always go back to the question and make sure you're choosing an answer that actually answers the question and is not just a true statement. An answer can be factually correct, but it MUST answer the question asked. Additionally, two answers can both be seemingly correct, so be sure to read all of the answer choices, and make sure that you get the one that BEST answers the question.

Milk the Question

Some of the questions may throw you completely off. They might deal with a subject you have not been exposed to, or one that you haven't reviewed in years. While your lack of knowledge about the subject will be a hindrance, the question itself can give you many clues that will help you find the correct answer. Read the question carefully and look for clues. Watch particularly for adjectives and nouns describing difficult terms or words that you don't recognize. Regardless of if you completely understand a word or not, replacing it with a synonym either provided or one you more familiar with may help you to understand what the questions are asking. Rather than wracking your mind about specific detailed information concerning a difficult term or word, try to use mental substitutes that are easier to understand.

The Trap of Familiarity

Don't just choose a word because you recognize it. On difficult questions, you may not recognize a number of words in the answer choices. The test writers don't put "make-believe" words on the test; so don't think that just because you only recognize all the words in one answer choice means that answer choice must be correct. If you only recognize words in one answer choice, then focus on that one. Is it correct? Try your best to determine if it is correct. If it is, that is great, but if it doesn't, eliminate it. Each word and answer choice you eliminate increases your chances of getting the question correct, even if you then have to guess among the unfamiliar choices.

Eliminate Answers

Eliminate choices as soon as you realize they are wrong. But be careful! Make sure you consider all of the possible answer choices. Just because one appears right, doesn't mean that the next one won't be even better! The test writers will usually put more than one good answer choice for every question, so read all of them. Don't worry if you are stuck between two that seem right. By getting down to just two remaining possible choices, your odds are now 50/50. Rather than wasting too much time, play the odds. You are guessing, but guessing wisely, because you've been able to knock out some of the answer choices that you know are wrong. If you are eliminating choices and realize that the last answer choice you are left with is also obviously wrong, don't panic. Start over and consider each choice again. There may easily be something that you missed the first time and will realize on the second pass.

Tough Questions

If you are stumped on a problem or it appears too hard or too difficult, don't waste time. Move on! Remember though, if you can quickly check for obviously incorrect answer choices, your chances of guessing correctly are greatly improved. Before you completely give up, at least try to knock out a couple of possible answers. Eliminate what you can and then guess at the remaining answer choices before moving on.

Brainstorm

If you get stuck on a difficult question, spend a few seconds quickly brainstorming. Run through the complete list of possible answer choices. Look at each choice and ask yourself, "Could this answer the question satisfactorily?" Go through each answer choice and consider it independently of the other. By systematically going through all possibilities, you may find something that you would otherwise overlook. Remember that when you get stuck, it's important to try to keep moving.

Read Carefully

Understand the problem. Read the question and answer choices carefully. Don't miss the question because you misread the terms. You have plenty of time to read each question thoroughly and make sure you understand what is being asked. Yet a happy medium must be attained, so don't waste too much time. You must read carefully, but efficiently.

Face Value

When in doubt, use common sense. Always accept the situation in the problem at face value. Don't read too much into it. These problems will not require you to make huge leaps of logic. The test writers aren't trying to throw you off with a cheap trick. If you have to go beyond creativity and make a leap of logic in order to have an answer choice answer the question, then you should look at the other answer choices. Don't overcomplicate the problem by creating theoretical relationships or explanations that will warp time or space. These are normal problems rooted in reality. It's just that the applicable relationship or explanation may not be readily apparent and you have to figure things out. Use your common sense to interpret anything that isn't clear.

Prefixes

If you're having trouble with a word in the question or answer choices, try dissecting it. Take advantage of every clue that the word might include. Prefixes and suffixes can be a huge help. Usually they allow you to determine a basic meaning. Pre- means before, post- means after, pro - is positive, de- is negative. From these prefixes and suffixes, you can get an idea of the general meaning of the word and try to put it into context. Beware though of any traps. Just because con is the opposite of pro, doesn't necessarily mean congress is the opposite of progress!

Hedge Phrases

Watch out for critical "hedge" phrases, such as likely, may, can, will often, sometimes, often, almost, mostly, usually, generally, rarely, sometimes. Question writers insert these hedge phrases to cover every possibility. Often an answer choice will be wrong simply because it leaves no room for exception. Avoid answer choices that have definitive words like "exactly," and "always".

Switchback Words

Stay alert for "switchbacks". These are the words and phrases frequently used to alert you to shifts in thought. The most common switchback word is "but". Others include although, however, nevertheless, on the other hand, even though, while, in spite of, despite, regardless of.

New Information

Correct answer choices will rarely have completely new information included. Answer choices typically are straightforward reflections of the material asked about and will directly relate to the question. If a new piece of information is included in an answer choice that doesn't even seem to relate to the topic being asked about, then that answer choice is likely incorrect. All of the information needed to answer the question is usually provided for you, and so you should not have to make guesses that are unsupported or choose answer choices that require unknown information that cannot be reasoned on its own.

Time Management

On technical questions, don't get lost on the technical terms. Don't spend too much time on any one question. If you don't know what a term means, then since you don't have a dictionary, odds are you aren't going to get much further. You should immediately recognize terms as whether or not you know them. If you don't, work with the other clues that you have, the other answer choices and terms provided, but don't waste too much time trying to figure out a difficult term.

Contextual Clues

Look for contextual clues. An answer can be right but not correct. The contextual clues will help you find the answer that is most right and is correct. Understand the context in which a phrase or statement is made. This will help you make important distinctions.

Don't Panic

Panicking will not answer any questions for you. Therefore, it isn't helpful. When you first see the question, if your mind goes blank, take a deep breath. Force yourself to mechanically go through the steps of solving the problem and using the strategies you've learned.

Pace Yourself

Don't get clock fever. It's easy to be overwhelmed when you're looking at a page full of questions, your mind is full of random thoughts and feeling confused, and the clock is ticking down faster than you would like. Calm down and maintain the pace that you have set for yourself. As long as you are on track by monitoring your pace, you are guaranteed to have enough time for yourself. When you get to the last few minutes of the test, it may seem like you won't have enough time left, but if you only have as many questions as you should have left at that point, then you're right on track!

Answer Selection

The best way to pick an answer choice is to eliminate all of those that are wrong, until only one is left and confirm that is the correct answer. Sometimes though, an answer choice may immediately look right. Be careful! Take a second to make sure that the other choices are not equally obvious. Don't make a hasty mistake. There are only two times that you should stop before checking other answers. First is when you are positive that the answer choice you have selected is correct. Second is when time is almost out and you have to make a quick guess!

Check Your Work

Since you will probably not know every term listed and the answer to every question, it is important that you get credit for the ones that you do know. Don't miss any questions through careless mistakes. If at all possible, try to take a second to look back over your answer selection and make sure you've selected the correct answer choice and haven't made a costly careless mistake (such as marking an answer choice that you didn't mean to mark). This quick double check should more than pay for itself in caught mistakes for the time it costs.

Beware of Directly Quoted Answers

Sometimes an answer choice will repeat word for word a portion of the question or reference section. However, beware of such exact duplication – it may be a trap! More than likely, the correct choice will paraphrase or summarize a point, rather than being exactly the same wording.

Slang

Scientific sounding answers are better than slang ones. An answer choice that begins "To compare the outcomes..." is much more likely to be correct than one that begins "Because some people insisted..."

Extreme Statements

Avoid wild answers that throw out highly controversial ideas that are proclaimed as established fact. An answer choice that states the "process should be used in certain situations, if..." is much

- 158 -

more likely to be correct than one that states the "process should be discontinued completely."   The first is a calm rational statement and doesn't even make a definitive, uncompromising stance, using a hedge word "if" to provide wiggle room, whereas the second choice is a radical idea and far more extreme.

Answer Choice Families

When you have two or more answer choices that are direct opposites or parallels, one of them is usually the correct answer. For instance, if one answer choice states "x increases" and another answer choice states "x decreases" or "y increases," then those two or three answer choices are very similar in construction and fall into the same family of answer choices. A family of answer choices is when two or three answer choices are very similar in construction, and yet often have a directly opposite meaning. Usually the correct answer choice will be in that family of answer choices. The "odd man out" or answer choice that doesn't seem to fit the parallel construction of the other answer choices is more likely to be incorrect.

Additional Bonus Material

Due to our efforts to try to keep this book to a manageable length, we've created a link that will give you access to all of your additional bonus material.

Please visit http://www.mometrix.com/bonus948/pmhn to access the information.

DISCARD

Made in the USA
Columbia, SC
21 July 2017